FALSE POSITIVE

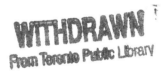

FALSE POSITIVE

Private Profit in
Canada's Medical Laboratories

Ross Sutherland

Fernwood Publishing • Halifax and Winnipeg

To our grandchildren Brianna and Ronnie, in the hope that we may find a way to build a community for them that serves human needs rather than private greed.

Editing and design: Brenda Conroy
Cover design: John van der Woude
Printed and bound in Canada by Hignell Book Printing

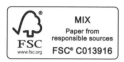

Published in Canada by Fernwood Publishing
32 Oceanvista Lane
Black Point, Nova Scotia, B0J 1B0
and 748 Broadway Avenue, Winnipeg, Manitoba, R3G 0X3
www.fernwoodpublishing.ca

Fernwood Publishing Company Limited gratefully acknowledges the financial support of the Government of Canada through the Canada Book Fund, the Canada Council for the Arts, the Nova Scotia Department of Tourism and Culture and the Province of Manitoba, through the Book Publishing Tax Credit, for our publishing program.

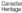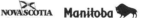

Library and Archives Canada Cataloguing in Publication

Sutherland, Ross, 1952-
  False positive : private profit in Canada's medical laboratories / Ross Sutherland.

(Basics)
Includes bibliographical references.
ISBN 978-1-55266-409-4

1. Medical laboratories--Canada. 2. Privatization.
I. Title. II. Series: Fernwood basics

R860.S87 2011   344.71'0547   C2010-908057-2

Contents

Acronyms

AHS — Alberta Health Services Board

AO — Archives of Ontario

BCMA — British Columbia Medical Association.

CMA — Canadian Medical Association

CMAJ — Canadian Medical Association Journal.

CML — Canadian Medical Laboratories before 2004 and after 2004 the CML Healthcare Fund — one of the largest for-profit laboratory providers in Canada, based primarily in Ontario.

CPSO — College of Physicians and Surgeons of Ontario — the institution charged with protecting the public from unethical and professional misconduct by physicians.

DKML — Dynacare Kasper Medical Laboratories.

DSM — Diagnostic Services of Manitoba

EORLA — Eastern Ontario Regional Laboratory Association

GDML — Gamma-Dynacare Medical Laboratories — one of Canada's largest for-profit medical laboratory companies and a subsidiary of the Laboratory Corporation of America, LabCorp.

HICL — Hospitals In-Common Laboratory.

HIDSA — Hospital Insurance and Diagnostic Services Act — federal legislation passed in 1958 and adopted in Ontario in 1959, which set up a cost-sharing program for the provision of hospital services.

HHSLP — Hamilton Health Science Laboratory Program — a regional laboratory program started in 1972, run by Hamilton hospitals and also provided community laboratory services.

HSRC — Hospital Services Restructuring Commission — a commission created in Ontario by the Harris Conservative government in 1996 to consolidate hospital services including their laboratories, chaired by Duncan Sinclair.

LHIN — Local Health Integration Network — Ontario's regional health care administrative body, established in 2004, which has jurisdiction over hospital laboratories but not over community laboratories.

LIS — Laboratory Information System.

LMS — labour, materials, and supervision — A system of workload measurement developed in Ontario for the community laboratories based on these factors. An LMS unit refers to the minimum unit of payment in the community laboratory sector and each test is assigned a number of LMS units.

LOPPP — Laboratory Outpatient Pilot Program — a pilot program in Ontario in 1981 to fund hospitals to provide community laboratory services.

LPTP — Laboratory Proficiency Testing Program — a program established by the Ontario government in 1974 and run by the OMA to monitor and improve quality in medical laboratories.

LSR — Laboratory Services Review — a review of laboratory services commissioned by Ontario's Bob Rae NDP government in 1992.

MDS — One of the largest for-profit laboratory corporations in Canada, bought in 2007 by the Ontario Municipal Employees Pension Plan and renamed LifeLabs.

MOH — Ministry of Health — used as a short hand to refer to the Ministry in the government of Ontario that has responsibility for medical laboratories. It is currently called the Ministry of Health and Long-term Care and started out as the Department of Health in the 1960s.

OAML — Ontario Association of Medical Laboratories — the organization representing the commercial laboratories.

OHA — Ontario Hospital Association.

OHIP — Ontario Health Insurance Plan — formed in 1972 by a merger of the insurance administrative structures of OHSC and OHSIP. In popular use OHIP has two meanings. It refers to the health insurance plan that covers all residents in Ontario, and it refers to the payment plan within the Ministry of Health that only covers medical services. Hospital services are insured through OHIP but paid for under a separate budget within a different department within the Ministry.

OHSC — Ontario Hospital Services Commission — set up to run hospital insurance in Ontario under the *HIDSA*.

OHSIP — Ontario Health Services Insurance Plan — formed in 1969 in response to the federal Medicare Act, it took over from OMSIP. OHSIP and the OHSC merged in 1972 to form OHIP.

OMA — Ontario Medical Association — the organization representing physicians.

OMSIP–Ontario Medical Service Insurance Plan — a voluntary medical services insurance plan set up by the provincial government in 1966, in part an attempt to prevent the movement towards a universal medical insurance plan, which ran until OHSIP was established in 1969.

ORLSP — Ontario Regional Laboratory Services Planning — a program begun in 2001 to facilitate regional plans for laboratory integration.

PPAC — Planning and Program Advisory Committee — an internal MOH committee in the mid-1970s.

PSI — Physicians' Services Incorporated — a non-profit medical insurance company set up in 1947 by the Ontario Medical Association.

QMP–LS — Quality Management Program–Laboratory Services — the quality assurance program that took over from the LPTP in 2000.

RFP — Request for Proposals.

RSC — Regional Steering Committee — the name of the regional coordinating body under the ORLSP.

SCC — Specimen Collection Centre — a place where laboratory specimens are taken, sometimes called bleeding stations.

TML — Toronto Medical Laboratory

UHN — University Hospital Network, consisting of the Toronto General, the Toronto Western and the Princess Margaret Hospitals.

Medical Laboratories and the Public-Private Debate

I first became aware that something was seriously wrong in our medical laboratory system in the 1990s while working as a home care nurse in eastern Ontario. I was part of a team administering intravenous antibiotics in patients' homes. Occasionally a patient exhibited dangerous symptoms that might have been a reaction to the drug; in these cases a prompt analysis of blood levels of the drug was required. MDS, a for-profit multinational health care corporation, had been awarded the contract to provide laboratory services to home care patients in Kingston, but using MDS meant sending the blood sample to Toronto for analysis. Some of these tests are uncommon, and often we would not get a result for a few days. This was unacceptable. We had to know whether or not it was safe to give the next dose later that day. So we simply sent the blood to the local hospital laboratory, where processing was done quickly and results were immediately available.

Unfortunately, because of government policy, the hospital received no money for providing this clearly superior service. Instead the service was paid for out of its general operating budget, reducing the funds available for other in-hospital services. MDS was unhappy because we were taking lucrative fee-for-service work away from them. The home care agency, the Community Care Access Centre, was unhappy because we were breaking the rules and, in our own small way, sabotaging the for-profit delivery of health services. But the nurses, patients and doctors were happy because we got the results we needed when we needed them.

Laboratories are central to the practice of mainstream medicine in Canada. They play a role in 80 percent of medical diagnoses. Most Canadians have had at least one intimate relationship with a medical laboratory in their lifetime, probably many more. Newborn babies have mandatory blood tests, children have their throats swabbed, healthy adults have stool and blood screening, and anyone with a significant illness has bodily fluids and/or tissue samples analyzed. In each instance, a wrong laboratory result can have dire consequences.

The last decade has seen a series of scandals involving the incorrect interpretation of women's pathology tests, a laboratory test to identify abnormalities in cells. The results were missed breast cancer diagnoses and incorrectly identified cancers. These laboratory errors caused many women to receive dangerous treatments they did not need and many others to be denied lifesaving treatment they did need. Many of the women affected did not live long enough to receive the compensation and apologies they deserved.

These tragic cases illustrate how important laboratory testing is. An incorrect drug screening test can cost a worker their job. A mislabelled blood sample could result in the administration of blood thinners to the wrong patient, increasing the risk of a stroke. An improperly collected or stored bacterial culture can result in an effective antibiotic treatment being delayed. Failure to collect water samples properly or report results, as happened in Walkerton Ontario, can result in serious harm to thousands of people. Yet labs tend to receive only passing mention in discussions of our health care system.

That the laboratory sector maintains a low profile is all the more surprising given the centrality of the services it provides. Laboratory workers comprise the third largest group of health care professionals, and medical laboratories consume over $4 billion of public money every year. Laboratory services have been called the touchstone of modern medical practice. Laboratory results are key to medical authority and foundational to medicine's evolution.

And labs are not strangers to controversy. There are regular accusations of fraud, over use, excessive cost and medical misconduct levelled against laboratories, but generally speaking what happens to our blood, sputum, stool or tissue samples after they leave our bodies does not concern us. Laboratory services are accepted as an integral, yet hidden, part of our health care system. Most people give little thought to who owns the labs, how their services are paid for, how they are organized or how the delivery of these services affects our public health care system. These services are unique among the key elements of our public acute care system in that for-profit multinational corporations play a central role in their delivery.

While largely unnoticed, for-profit medical laboratories have not been absent from the debate on the future of medicare. Their existence has been used to argue that greater private involvement in our health care system is more efficient and effective than relying on non-profit public services. Contrary to these arguments, which are driven by a naive belief in the superiority of markets and the profit motive, this book shows that in the case of Canada's medical laboratory services, the exclusive use of public, non-profit organizations would be the best way to increase access, control costs, integrate services, improve quality and enhance the democratic control of health care.

The Public-Private Debate

One of the central policy debates in Canada is over the future of universal health care for medically necessary services. Although medicare continues to enjoy enormous popular support (IPSOS 2006), as it has since its inception, it is under attack. This is not surprising. Health care in Canada is big business, as it is in most advanced capitalist countries. Canada's total yearly public expenditure on health care is approximately $135 billion; it accounts for over 40 percent of Ontario program spending. Robert Evans, writing in 1993, commented tongue-in-cheek, "there has always been a crisis in Canadian health care," (35) and the reasons are always the same: cutbacks, shortages and spiralling costs. The main perpetrators of this crisis rhetoric continue to be those who wish to lower the costs to the "wealthy and healthy" and increase the benefits to the for-profit health care corporations.

These threats to our public health care system are being challenged by a broad-based coalition of community and labour organizations, whose members argue that our current system is sustainable, provides security for citizens and embodies what is best about social reform: it is inclusive and collective and it places need before ability to pay. Universal health care is essential to a functioning democracy (Leys 2001).

While the main issue in these debates is often universal public insurance for essential health care services, the question, as Robert Evans (1997) notes, is really closed: most observers in health policy and political circles agree medicare is more cost-effective and efficient than the alternatives. Even ideological free market supporters, such as Prime Minister Steven Harper, have stopped directly attacking universal health insurance.

There is less unanimity on the question of private delivery. Private corporate interests have increased their pressure for more for-profit clinics to provide a variety of services: MRIs and CT scans, cataract surgeries, joint replacements, family medical services, home care and the construction and operation of hospitals. Armine Yalnizyan (2004) identifies the growing use of public funds to pay for private, for-profit delivery of services as one of the four main threats to the sustainability of Canada's public health care system.

The history of the development of medical laboratory services in Canada goes to the heart of the debate on the private delivery of publicly insured medical services. In medical laboratories, we have a forty-year case study on the use of for-profit companies to provide an essential medical service. The results are clear: these companies are more expensive and they have fought integration, undercut democracy and negatively impacted access and quality in our health care system. They are a threat to the sustainability of universal health care.

A study of Canada's community laboratory services provides a comparison between non-profit institutions and private corporations in the delivery of the same service. The evolution of community laboratory services is the story of the development of three multinational health service corporations — MDS/LifeLabs, CML and Dynacare — and the intentional undermining of public, non-profit laboratory services.

This analysis takes seriously Colin Leys' admonition: "the impacts of economic forces need to be studied not only at the level of politics in general but also in specific markets" (2001: 81): in this case the public market for medical laboratory services.

Medical laboratories started as non-profit facilities in our public health services and the public hospital system. After the introduction of medicare in 1968, for-profit laboratory corporations expanded rapidly in five provinces.

Government policies created a market for their services, public money funded their growth, and institutions were established to consolidate their political power. Government policy in favour of the greater use of private laboratories was strongly supported by actions of the medical profession.

The structure of Canadian federalism provides a national and provincial context for exploring the specific impacts of changes in global capitalism on Canada's community laboratory services. The shift to a more corporate laboratory service paralleled the development of global capital markets and the rise of neoliberalism as a political project to undercut collective services, such as health care, and increase opportunities for private profit. The publicly funded development of commercial laboratories has also increased international economic integration by both facilitating the expansion of Canadian companies onto the international stage and allowing American capital to buy into Canada.

What Is Public and What Is Private?

Discussion of the use of private corporations is made more difficult both by terminology and by the reality of the Canadian health care system. The fact that Canada's health care system is a mix of for-profit, non-profit and public is obvious. Many private, for-profit companies, such as laboratory giants LifeLabs (formerly MDS), Gamma-Dynacare and Canadian Medical Laboratories (CML), make the bulk of their money from public funds and often do not charge patients directly for their services. On the other hand, hospitals are legally private, non-profit corporations that regularly contract out some of their services to for-profit companies and occasionally charge patients directly for care. This blurring of the lines between the public and private reflects the penetration of the market into this core government program. It muddies the waters of popular debate and is often used as a lever to increase market involvement. How the terms *public* and *private* are used is as much a political matter as a semantic one.

Most Canadians perceive public health care services to be those they receive as a right of citizenship under the *Canada Health Act*; this includes most laboratory services. While this perception is helpful in maintaining broad access and support for universal health insurance, it hides questions of ownership and control: a bias reflecting capitalist societies' tendency to focus on individual consumers rather than the social system of production.

The confusion is reinforced by a classification system common among academics that uses a juridical approach to categorize health care institutions as either public, those directly part of the civil service, or private, including non-profit hospitals, doctors and for-profit providers (Deber 2004). While the governance structure of institutions can be important, in this context the classification is often used to undercut the progressive use of the term "privatization" because it defines most current health care delivery as private, making privatization a non-issue. Duncan Sinclair, former chair of Ontario's Health Service Restructuring Commission, used this approach in a CBC radio interview on March 29, 2007 to downplay the significance of moving ancillary services out of hospitals. The governance approach also ignores the increasing centralization of health care decision-making in most provinces; hospitals and other health services are coming more and more under direct government control, regardless of their legal incorporation.

A distinction central to this book, one that is important to understanding our medical laboratory system and crucial to the future of our health care system, is the distinction between corporations that operate for private profit and providers that are non-profit, operating within some broadly defined notion of public good. In this book, references to private labs and other private health care services are references to for-profit corporations, i.e., companies that need to pay dividends to their investors.

Non-profit entities include those run directly by the government as well as non-profit corporations such as hospitals, the Victorian Order of Nurses, community health centres and the Centre Local de Services Communautaires in Quebec. While there are significant differences within this group, they share a primary interest in delivering health care for collective benefit rather than to make a return on investment. Profit is not part of their decision-making equation.

One group that is central to the story of the for-profit laboratories does not neatly fit into this dichotomy: unincorporated private practice physicians. Most likely, the goals of most of these practitioners are to maximize their personal income within the funding incentives, deliver a service and pay their bills. There are, of course, some who use their position as a springboard to corporate medicine and the exploitation of insurance schemes for extraordinary private gain and power. This practice is very evident in the history of private laboratories. There are, for example, the cases of Dr. John Mull, a pathologist who parlayed his practice into Canadian Medical Laboratories, Dr. T.A. Kasper, who founded Kasper Laboratories in Alberta, and Dr. Cam Coady and the consortium of pathologists who founded BC Biomedical laboratories.

The dynamic of turning their profession into an investment opportunity continues with the likes of Doctors Brian Day and Robert Ouellet, both recent past presidents of the Canadian Medical Association, who used their medical credentials to found for-profit corporations and make significant amounts of money from the public purse. It is a predictable outcome of the individual autonomous practice model dominant among Canadian physicians.

Doctors as a group have also used their influence to systematically work against public, non-profit options, whether fighting universal health insurance, demanding the right to extra-bill patients or calling for more innovation (for which read: more for-profit participation) in the Canadian health care system. One lesson from the evolution of laboratory services is that private practice physicians who bill fee-for-service are more likely to challenge the collective provision of health care than those primarily associated with public hospitals, who are much more likely to support a universal, integrated, accessible health care system.

How Medical Laboratories Work

To understand the political economy of Canada's medical laboratory industry it helps to have a general knowledge of how patients are classified and what the key components of the medical laboratory system are. A central concern in policy debates on medical laboratories is how services are provided to different types of patients. Three common classifications of patients are: inpatients, who are assigned a bed in a hospital; outpatients, who receive medical services in a hospital but are not assigned a bed; and community patients, who receive medical services in the community, most often from a family physician. For the purposes of this book, patients are usually divided into only two groups: inpatients, who receive their laboratory services while staying in the hospital, paid for out of the hospital's budget; and community patients, including both outpatients and community patients, who may, depending on the province, have the option of having their laboratory work done in a hospital or by a for-profit corporation. The primary debate on for-profit provision of laboratory work focuses on how and where community patients should have their samples processed and how these should be paid for.

Schematically, laboratory work consists of taking a sample, transporting it to a lab, analyzing it and conveying useful results back to the health care provider and patient. Since most samples are small they can easily be transported to a facility for evaluation. The path a sample takes depends upon the patient, the laboratory and the professionals involved. Patients in hospitals usually have their blood taken by a nurse and then it is sent to an on-site laboratory for processing. The results and interpretation are quickly available to the attending medical staff. Patients in the community often have their blood taken in a specimen collection centre (SCC), or bleeding station, often located in a building that also houses doctors. Most of these samples are transported to a central processing facility, usually in another city. Fax, mail, phone and computer are used to inform the physician of the results. Another option, both in hospitals and the community, is point-of-care testing, in which a sample is tested in a doctor's office or at the bedside. The relationships between specimen collection, testing, reporting and interpreting are more complicated than these simple schemata suggest. But how these basic elements are delivered, financed and coordinated are the central concerns of medical laboratory policy considered in this book.

An important aspect of medical laboratory work not covered in this book is public health services. This decision was made primarily for space reasons. Public health laboratories provide an invaluable public service but account for less than 5 percent of laboratory expenses, and to do justice to some of the complexities in their development would have taken more pages than are possible in this volume.

Most data in this book come from research for my master's thesis on the political economy of Ontario's medical laboratory industry (Sutherland 2007). The findings rely on extensive research in the Archives of Ontario and on confidential interviews with key informants. Ontario also occupies a large space in this book because the corporations that dominate private medical laboratory services in Canada have their roots in Ontario. The policies of successive Ontario governments, of all political stripes, under the rubric of public medical and hospital insurance, have allowed these companies to flourish. Understanding this process in Ontario helps one to understand many of the developments that have taken place in other provinces.

Fifty years ago most community specimens were analyzed by public institutions (hospitals and public health laboratories) or by doctors in private practice. Today, in many provinces, for-profit corporations play a significant role. This transformation has been particularly profound in Ontario, where over 90 percent of community lab services are provided by three multinationals.

Cost and Integration

This book evaluates the impact of for-profit corporations on the delivery of laboratory services, focusing on system cost and integration. Reducing the cost of laboratory services has been a central policy goal of all provinces with for-profit laboratories since the introduction of medicare. This study is restricted to the cost to the government of providing medically necessary laboratory services. It does not include, for instance, other social costs incurred by using for-profit companies, e.g., workers who are paid less or costs to smaller communities as a result of having laboratory services centralized in a few large population centres. While these are important societal considerations and need to be studied, they are outside the scope of this book. This book does not simply assume that cost reduction is the ultimate good. Clearly, there are other social goals that would justify a government choosing more expensive alternatives. Providing adequate pay and working conditions, good access for all patients and superior quality easily come to mind.

Along with cost control, the integration of laboratory services has been a key policy objective of all provincial governments; the Ontario government has had this objective since 1960. In this book integration is usually used in the positive sense of maximizing the efficient use of resources and, from the patients' perspective, of coordination for improved quality and accessibly. But integration is not an unqualified good. Centralizing services can decrease access, hurt the ability of smaller community hospitals to provide basic laboratory services and decrease quality of care by creating barriers between practising physicians and laboratory specialists. The interactions between resources spent on services, their quality, accessibility and democracy are an important part of this story. For example, quality considerations were central to early initiatives by governments to regulate private corporations and played a role in their consolidation.

A reason to focus on cost is that supporters of more for-profit involvement in laboratory services claim that it will reduce cost. In essence this is a critique of that position. Cost control and integration of laboratory services are two policy prescriptions with broad support across the country, and yet they have never been successfully implemented. The focus on cost and integration also provides an opening through which we can explore an alternative approach to understanding government policy, the interaction of governments with for-profit providers and the struggle over resources at the centre of the analysis.

This study of Canada's medical laboratory services pays special attention to three themes important to understanding how a few small for-profit laboratories led to the rise of multinational for-profit laboratory corporations. The first theme is the interactions between for-profit corporations and government, both in terms of how governments have favoured these services and how companies have influenced decision-making. The second theme covers how the medical profession, and more broadly the practice of biomedicine, has been instrumental in setting the conditions for private delivery, giving it legitimacy and covering up its failings. Third, we look at changes in laboratory policy over the last forty years, which provides insights into how changes in the global economy impact the delivery of local services.

Outline of the Book

The first chapter describes the development of a strong national non-profit laboratory system before the *Medical Care Act* of 1968 and some of the influences, largely from the medical community, that limited its reach and laid the basis for the development of a for-profit sector. These non-profit services were primarily delivered through public health departments and in hospitals, which continue to be the backbone of our medical laboratory system.

Chapter Two examines the changes in Ontario government policy from 1968 to 1990 that facilitated the rise of for-profit laboratory corporations from the few small private labs that were allowed to exist before medicare. At the same time that Ontario's Conservative governments were establishing structures that facilitated for-profit growth, they were concerned about this expansion. Chapter Three describes the support given in Ontario to non-profit community laboratory services. Compared to private laboratories, these public sector organizations were better able to control costs and improve service integration.

Chapter Four examines the developments in laboratory services in Ontario from 1990 to 2010. During this period we saw the height of neoliberal influence. The federal government reduced funding to provinces for health care, and the NDP government in Ontario, faced with a recession and escalating public debt, negotiated directly with the for-profit laboratory companies to cut provincial payments for laboratory services. The trade-off was increased control and financial security for the large private laboratories.

Chapter Five provides descriptions of the three largest for-profit laboratory corporations in Canada — LifeLabs (formerly MDS), Canadian Medical Laboratories (CML) and Gamma-Dynacare, a wholly owned subsidiary of the second largest laboratory services corporation in the United States, the Laboratory Corporation of America (LabCorp) — and what they have done with our health care dollars. The genesis of all three can be directly traced back to the corporatization of private doctors' practices.

Chapter Six outlines medical laboratory services in the other nine provinces, focusing on connections between funding, ownership and delivery. Six provinces, British Columbia to Quebec, use a mix of public and private laboratories for community patients. There has recently been a small move away from using for-profit corporations; instead governments have been focusing on restructuring non-profit services along "business lines," hampering the delivery of public laboratory services and possibly easing the way for more privatization in the future.

Chapter Seven addresses the argument that for-profit laboratories have been so successful because they provide more cost-effective service and help meet governmental goals of greater service integration. While problems of business secrecy and structural differences between hospital and community laboratory systems make direct comparisons difficult, the arguments and available data make a compelling case that for-profit laboratory services cost at least 25 percent more than using non-profit institutions. As well as being more expensive, private corporations have played an active role in undercutting integration initiatives. Using a fully integrated non-profit laboratory system to deliver all services would likely save the Canadian health care system at least $250 million in 2010.

Chapter Eight continues to challenge the argument that for-profit companies provide a better service by considering the effects of using these corporations on quality and access. Chapter Nine returns to the debate on the use of for-profit corporations to deliver publicly funded health care. The history of laboratory services in Canada provides evidence that for-profit delivery works against the sustainability, accessibility, quality and democratic control of our public health care system. It is recommended that fee-for-service payments for laboratory services be ended and that a transition to a fully integrated public non-profit laboratory service begin.

Chapter 1

Medical Laboratory Services before Medicare

Securing a Strong Non-Profit Sector

Modern medical laboratories services have their roots in the public health movement of the nineteenth century. Building on scientific discoveries in bacteriology and using relatively simple technologies, medical laboratories quickly gained a central place in the implementation of preventative measures, for example, improving sanitation and sexually transmitted disease identification and tracking. In 1884, the newly formed Ontario Provincial Board of Health established, on the grounds of the University of Toronto, one of the first public health laboratories in North America (Bator and Rhodes 1990).

Early public health efforts were complemented by laboratory services in a growing number of hospitals. These hospitals were funded by public revenues, community donations, patient payments and, as the twentieth century advanced, private insurance payments. Because of their financially precarious nature and their role in providing care to indigent populations, hospitals were formed as non-profit institutions. They were also designed to meet the medical community's need for training and, as medical science improved, to be a place where more expensive technologies could be purchased, made available to medical staff and accessed by those who could afford them (Swartz 1977: 328).The following personal account describes the development of laboratory services in a northwestern Ontario community:

> Our first Hospital Laboratory was equipped by Medical Staff, [and] the Hospital grudgingly giving us, about 1932, a room four by ten. A little later the Hospital employed one technician and she was given a room 10 x10 with minimum equipment..... During these latter years Blue Cross started to pay the Hospitals for Laboratory service and then the use rapidly developed. [These developments complemented an] excellent Provincial [public health] Laboratory at Fort William…. This Laboratory has had a continuous record of service since 1919.[1]

Hospital and public health laboratories started as public, non-profit services because they were designed to fulfill social needs that could not be easily turned into profit-making opportunities (Leys 2009).

After the Second World War, the federal government provided grants to the provinces to build more hospitals. This was a mixed blessing for provincial coffers. While it established a network of non-profit community-based hospitals in all regions of Canada, it also added significantly to local and provincial financial troubles since many hospitals regularly ran deficits. Federal grants were also provided to expand diagnostic services, specifically to buy equipment, expand facilities and train workers.[2] These grants were only available to non-profit programs.

In the post-war period there was increased public pressure for access to the expanding hospital and diagnostic services. This pressure, plus the example of the successful universal hospital insurance programs in British Columbia and Saskatchewan and the increased demands from the provinces for more financial assistance, lead to the passage of the *Hospital Insurance and Diagnostic Services Act* (HIDSA) in 1957 (Taylor 1978).HIDSA established a cost-sharing program between the federal and provincial governments to pay for a national non-profit hospital system and access for all Canadians to a full range of inpatient hospital care. To receive federal money hospitals were expected to provide good quality diagnostic services. The term "diagnostic services" refers to both laboratory and radiological services. HIDSA came into force in Ontario in 1959.

By the 1960s public money and programs had established a network of non-profit laboratory services across Canada to meet the needs of both inpatients and community patients. But there were limitations on these services as a result of opposition from powerful special interest groups, notably doctors and private insurance companies.

Non-Profit Hospital Insurance, Doctors and Laboratory Services

The medical profession, led by radiologists and pathologists, was the main opposition to a national hospital insurance program and an integrated system of laboratory services (Taylor 1978: 219). On top of their antipathy to "state medicine," pathologists were particularly concerned about proposals to provide outpatient diagnostic services in public facilities. This would limit their growing private business of providing laboratory services.

The initial federal and provincial proposals on national hospital insurance included outpatient diagnostic services as a mandatory benefit. Malcolm Taylor writes: "The question of out-patient diagnostic services was to become a serious issue between the Government and the OMA [Ontario Medical Association]" (1978: 131). The OMA wanted diagnostic services to be treated differently from hospital services. The association considered it an affront that any medical service, including laboratory work, should be under the control of "lay" institutions, that is, hospitals, instead of being provided by independent medical practitioners. One pathologist, Dr. H.G. Pritzker, also argued that hospitals, like public health labs, would make it "exceedingly difficult" to run a private laboratory practice because in most parts of Canada provincial public health laboratories offered their services at "little or no cost to the physician and patient" (1957: 413). Pritzker proposed that the hospitals provide the space and equipment for diagnostic services and that pathologists would run the facilities and be paid on a fee-for-service basis for both inpatient and outpatient services. Health system

planners and hospital administrators were concerned that divesting management of laboratory services would lead to extra administrative work, the loss of
integrated medical services for inpatients and the loss of revenue from selling
laboratory services to community patients. They argued that diagnostics should
continue to be "part of a day of patient care" (Taylor 1978: 141).

HIDSA overrode some of the profession's concerns and made coverage of
diagnostic services for inpatients mandatory but left the provision of outpatient
services to provincial discretion. Ontario decided not to cover outpatient services, thus maintaining peace with the OMA. But with diagnostic services only
being covered for inpatients, the result was unnecessary hospital admissions to
access these services, which obviously involved extra costs (Taylor 1978). By
leaving a significant volume of work that could be performed by doctors, usually pathologists, in independent labs, this system also contributed greatly to
the emergence of private laboratory corporations. The medical lobby in Ontario
was successful in keeping outpatient diagnostic services out of the provincial
hospital insurance scheme until 1969. Mounting public dissatisfaction and the
introduction of universal medical insurance in 1968 changed hospital regulations
so that anyone requesting treatment at an outpatient department would not be
charged for most services; the costs would be covered either through the hospital
budget or billed back to the medical services insurance plan.[3] With outpatient
laboratory services covered, physicians, primarily pathologists, who already
had contracts with hospitals, started to bill separately for laboratory services;
this double billing escalated laboratory costs, medical costs and pathologists'
incomes.

The Medical Insurance Honey Pot

The 1950s saw an expansion in the number of non-governmental for-profit
and non-profit medical insurance plans covering the costs of doctors' services
outside hospitals. This growth was spurred by a desire to undercut increasing
public pressure for universal medical insurance and to provide assured payments
to doctors. It is unlikely that for-profit laboratories would have grown without
medical insurance to pay their bills and fund their profits.

Indeed, expenditures on laboratory services increased rapidly with the
expansion of medical insurance coverage. It is estimated that even before medicare, 90 to 95 percent of laboratory work was covered by medical insurance
(Chemical Engineering Research 1969).Physician Services Insurance (PSI), a
large non-profit insurer in Ontario founded after the Second World War and run
by the medical profession, reported that, "in 1962 costs [for laboratory service
claims] doubled, by 1964 they had more than doubled again, and between 1965
and 1968 costs quadrupled. The cost per participant per month in 1957 was a
third of a cent, and in 1968 it was 17 cents, an increase of more than 5000%"
(*Ontario Medical Review* 1969: 275).

The establishment in 1966 of a government-run voluntary insurance plan,
the Ontario Medical Services Insurance Plan (OMSIP), fed into the frenzy. The

director of the province's Laboratory Services Branch noted that within a year of the establishment of OMSIP, "private and commercial laboratories were mushrooming with thoughts of large assured profits."[4] A study of OMSIP billing data found that the utilization of commercial laboratories increased 225 percent from 1967 to 1968, compared with 104 percent for hospital outpatient billing and 97 percent for labs that were part of a doctor's practice (Boyd 1969).Of the 112 for-profit labs operating in Ontario in 1967, 15 percent were founded before 1950 while 50 percent were established between 1963 and 1967 (Chemical Engineering Research 1969: 7).   In 1966, Dr. K.C. Charron, Ontario deputy minister of health, responding to recommendations in the Laboratory Committee report, commented that, "private laboratories could most easily be controlled by refusal to provide public monies for laboratory work performed outside hospital or public health laboratories, which would be conducted at cost, removing any profit motive of quantity over quality."[5] Unfortunately, the Ontario government of the day did not follow this advice.

Insurance money also maintained physician control of the commercial enterprises. Before medicare, private insurance companies, notably the doctor-owned PSI, adopted a simple formula to determine which laboratories could be used for insured services: the laboratory had to be controlled by a licensed medical practitioner. The rationale for this approach is rooted in a central assumption of biomedicine: doctors, as medical authorities, would ensure that laboratories would only provide needed and quality services. It also added to the power and income of doctors.

To get around this formula, private laboratories would sometimes enter into arrangements of convenience; they would name a physician the "titular director" in order to be able to claim insurance funding (Chemical Engineering Research 1969).In a submission to the Committee on the Healing Arts, the managing director of the Doctors' Clinical Laboratory recounted how he, an entrepreneur, had set up a private clinical laboratory as an investment of private capital and hoped to make a profit.[6] He felt his service was well received by physicians but to keep his business from failing he had to transfer ownership to physicians. He advocated for non-medical business owners being able to receive insurance money to run a laboratory. Ironically, the OMA facilitated this transition in the 1970s.

Billing for Work Not Done

Doctors increased their earnings from laboratory services by structuring payments so that they were paid for work they did not do. Historically, physicians billed patients directly for their services, including laboratory work, and determined their own fees based upon a schedule set by the OMA. The assumption underlying the laboratory fee structure was that each test was done by a doctor, who was not only responsible for the result but did most of the work. Even at the turn of the twentieth century, in the earliest medical laboratories, this was a fiction (Twohig 2005). Doctors, usually male, hired laboratory assistants, usually female, to perform much of the work, which the doctors then took the credit and payment for. This division between work done and payment received was exacerbated by increased automation in the 1950s and 1960s. As the procedures became more automated, doctors played an ever smaller role in individual tests. Yet the fees paid assumed that a doctor, not a machine, was performing the test.

This problem was widely recognized. A 1969 study on private laboratories reported:

> There is very little doubt that the OMA Schedule of Fees gives quite a generous fee for the amount of work done. This is partially because the fee includes an allowance for interpretation by a pathologist and this interpretation does not normally take place. (Chemical Engineering Research 1969: 14)

The increased reliance on insurance payments, coupled with the increasing variety and volume of tests, gave insurers a significant interest in controlling the amount of the fees. This created a conundrum for PSI, the largest private insurance company in Ontario, because it was owned by the OMA. Controlling costs meant cutting the incomes of its members. In the end, PSI agreed to pay 90 percent of the OMA fee schedule, which doctors had set, and extra-billing, i.e., charging patients above this rate, for insured services was not allowed.[7]

In the early 1960s, the OMA responded to the reality of rapidly rising laboratory costs, which threatened to increase insurance premiums, by instructing the OMA tariff committee to consider separating the technical cost and the professional component in laboratory fees (*Ontario Medical Review* 1964). Initially, the committee responded by increasing the number of laboratory procedures that should be included within the fee for a normal visit to a doctor (*Ontario Medical Review* 1965).This produced a paradoxical effect. Physicians started to establish laboratories, but rather than run the tests themselves as part of their visit fee, they referred patients to their lab and had the lab bill for the test. In this way they received payment for both the visit and the test. As a result, the number of private laboratories increased, and so did the costs.

Summary

Before universal medical insurance, a collective social need for public health services and popular pressure for access to hospital services led to the creation of a national network of non-profit medical laboratories. The medical profession and entrepreneurs countered these progressive developments by restricting the scope of hospital insurance and working with early private medical insurance programs to reinforce the authority of doctors and create a network of private laboratories. The activities of these for-profit laboratories raised public concerns about unnecessary testing, fraud, reduced quality and uneven access to services. These emerging private laboratories were strengthened under universal medical insurance, which facilitated the eventual takeover of

Ontario's community laboratory services by corporate interests. This is the story in the next chapter.

Notes

1. Letter from Walter P. Hogarth to M. Dymond, Minister of Health, December 29, 1965. AO, RG 10-6-0-262, box 25, capitals in the original.
2. "Laboratory & Radiological Services," Committee on Federal Health Grants, January 8/54 and attachment "Laboratory and Radiological Services Grant," December 23, 1953. AO, RG 10 – 106, box 87.
3. "Commission Policies under the Global Budget System," memo from the OHSC Commission of Finance to Administrators of All Public Hospitals," July 7, 1970. AO, RG 10-1-2, file 1207.
4. "Laboratory Licensing: Background Information," report attached to a memo from W.J.A. Percy, Director, Laboratory Services Branch, to G.J. Chatfield, General Manger, Direct Services Division, Ministry of Health, September 12, 1973. AO, RG 10-39, box 3, B167577.
5. K.C. Charron, Deputy Minister of Health, letter to J.B. Neilson, Chairman, Ontario Hospital Services Commission, February 3, 1966. AO, RG 10-6-0-262, box 25.
6. J.C. MacLaurin, Managing Director of Doctors' Clinical Laboratory, "Brief for the Committee on the Health Arts: the views and Opinions of a Private Laboratory," undated. AO, RG 10-247-0-30, container 4, B134867.
7. Morton Schulman, MPP for High Park, Ontario Legislature, *Hansard*, May 7, 1968: 2603.

Chapter 2

The Rise of the For-Profits, 1968–1990

Ontario government policies in the decade after the introduction of medicare shaped the market for community laboratory services, funded the expansion of for-profit companies and drove their consolidation. The rise of these corporations took place despite a succession of government ministers, bureaucrats and health policy analysts who had serious concerns about private provision of community laboratory services. Robert Welsh, secretary for social development in the Conservative government in Ontario in 1972, expressed some of the concern: "We certainly need to prevent cost gouging... by private laboratories... in which medical practitioners often have a pecuniary interest."[1]

This chapter points to serious difficulties with the idea that private health care contractors can be easily controlled and that problems of over utilization, fraud, conflict of interest, poor quality and restricted access can be adequately mitigated. Even during the early 1970s — a time relatively favourable to collective solutions to health care needs, when a Conservative government had recently nationalized the bulk of the medical insurance industry and most bureaucrats in the Ministry of Health and most health policy analysts favoured increasing hospital laboratory use — for-profit corporations were able to overcome opposition, use regulations to their advantage and grow and prosper. Attempts made to direct work to hospital laboratories, encourage non-profit alternatives and limit the problems in for-profit provision of services were largely unsuccessful. Inherent biases in the capitalist state favouring private profit — business confidentiality, privileged political influence and unquestioned assumptions of market superiority — aided by the increasing power of private capital in the Canadian and world economies, thwarted the development of collective solutions to providing laboratory services.

Medicare and Increased Utilization

With the implementation of the national *Medical Care Insurance Act* (1966) in Ontario in 1969 all medically necessary services, including laboratory services, were covered by universal government insurance. The private laboratory industry, which already had a strong beachhead in Ontario, providing 8 percent of laboratory services in 1967 (Chemical Engineering Research 1969), took full advantage of this opening. Fee-for-service laboratory payments increased 25 percent from 1970 to 1971. And, while laboratory utilization increased in both the community and hospitals, community services rose significantly faster (Ontario Council 1982) and continued to increase until the Ontario government imposed hard caps on payments in 1993. A similar phenomenon occurred in

Table 2-1   Percent Increase in Laboratory Expenditure by Ownership,
1972–1991 (actual dollars)

	72–75	75–81	81–91
For-Profit	218%	67%	283%
Hospital	53%	54%	147%

Source: 1972–1981, Minster's Briefing Book: Laboratory Services Branch," May 21, 1985, p. 22.
AO, RG-39, box 5, B383120; 1991, (Ontario Ministry of Health 1993e).

British Columbia, Alberta and Saskatchewan, where the costs of fee-for-service laboratory work rose more rapidly than costs in the public sector, and often faster than total medical costs (Fagg et al. 1999; Bayne 2003; Kilshaw et al. 1992, also see Table 2.1).

It would be wrong to say that universal insurance was the only cause of increased utilization. Better medical science, new technologies, different tests, greater reliance on laboratory results, an increase in the number of doctors and a growing population were all part of the equation. But the spike after the introduction of medicare is unmistakable. And factors such as new tests, increased technology and more doctors were at least partially driven by the lure of ever-expanding fee-for-service income guaranteed by universal insurance.

Global Budgets and Limiting Hospital Access to OHIP Money

Even though inpatient laboratory costs rose less rapidly than community costs, hospital budgets were the first to be limited (Gold, Plant and MacKillop 1979). Ironically, two moves that helped control laboratory costs within hospitals, global budgets and limiting access to funds for outpatient services, increased the government's overall laboratory costs by transferring work to the for-profit companies.

The government introduced global budgets for hospitals in 1969. Global budgets fund hospitals with one payment for all the services instead of payments for each individual service. This lump sum payment is intended to give hospitals more flexibility to move money between programs to meet local needs in a cost-effective manner. The change to global budgets from line-by-line budgets was not specifically aimed at reducing the cost of diagnostic services — but it did have a significant effect on the provision of community laboratory services by hospitals.

After 1968, hospitals in Ontario were mandated to provide laboratory services to outpatients at no direct cost to the patient. As mentioned previously, this policy created unexpected financial opportunities for hospital physicians, primarily pathologists. Physicians who provided diagnostic services for outpatients were allowed to bill medicare on a fee-for-service basis while being paid a salary for providing inpatient pathology services and managing the hospitals' laboratories. The rapidly rising incomes of pathologists quickly become a political issue, and the government introduced regulations to stop hospital-based laboratory specialists from billing the medical insurance plan for outpatient laboratory services.

To further control hospital laboratory costs, in 1971 the Ontario Hospital Services Commission (OHSC) switched from fee-for-service payments to hospitals to a monthly bulk payment for outpatient laboratory services based on an estimate of outpatient work at 90 percent of the OMA fee schedule. "Considerable" savings were made in clerical costs due to the reduced paperwork.[2] Pathologists in hospitals were now only paid through their contractual agreement with the hospital; and, moving outpatient laboratory work to the institutional budget meant that the cost was shared with the federal government under *HIDSA*, a more lucrative formula for the province than the cost-sharing under the *Medical Care Act.*[3]

Then, as part of the anti-inflation constraints beginning in the late 1970s, top-up payments to hospitals for community laboratory work ended in 1980. Even though they were still legally obliged to provide laboratory services to community patients, doing so meant taking resources from other hospital programs covered by the global budget. With no incentive to provide service to community patients hospitals made no effort to attract this work. Ontario government policy had effectively secured the expanding community laboratory market for the for-profit corporations.

Direct Funding for Private Laboratories

When medicare was first introduced there was a significant barrier to the corporate takeover of the community laboratories. Under Ontario's early insurance schemes and then under Section 22(2) of the *Health Insurance Act* (1972), medicare payments could only be made for services "rendered by a physician," which in the case of laboratory services meant that doctors, usually pathologists, billed for all the work, including the less skilled technical that they did not perform. By 1971, the OMA fee schedule formally incorporated a lower technical fee for tests that did not involve any professional work, but there was little incentive for pathologists to bill only for the professional fee or not bill if they did not interpret the test. They argued that they should be paid both rates because they were responsible for the results.

As part of its efforts to control costs, the government overrode the pathologists' position and in 1973 amended the general regulation under the *Health Insurance Act* to allow licensed labs to bill OHIP directly for the technical component of laboratory work as long as it was ordered by a physician. This established a direct path for the commercial laboratories to medicare money. Since these technical fees were part of the OMA fee schedule, they were fee-for-service: the more tests commercial laboratories performed the higher their income. This fee structure formed a strong link between the labs and the family doctors. The laboratory companies needed the doctors to order higher volumes of tests to increase their income and profits. Laboratory medical specialists were only paid when they provided an interpretation and the laboratory corporation was paid for processing all the samples. In the short term, the OMA protected doctors' power and income by maintaining control of the technical and professional fees and ensuring that each laboratory had a doctor as medical director.

The division between global funding for hospitals and fee-for-service funding for community laboratories was reinforced by the establishment of a different workload measurement system for Ontario's community laboratories.

A Different Workload Measurement System

When laboratory technical and professional fees were established, as was the case with all other OMA rates, the individual services were simply assigned a monetary value. In 1973, the OMA and the Ministry entered into discussions to switch to a workload measurement system called LMS (labour, material and supervision) to arrive at a price for each laboratory test. Once the LMS unit value was set — how much labour, material and supervision was involved in each test — it would be multiplied by a negotiated figure to arrive at the amount paid for that test. When the system was introduced in 1974, the negotiated value of each LMS unit was 33 cents.[4]

Without an incredible amount of ongoing evaluation, it proved impossible for the LMS system to reflect new technologies, new testing procedures and changes in reagents and material handling systems. By 1976, it was understood that for commercial laboratories there was no "reliable" measure of the LMS units in each test and therefore no reliable data on which to determine the cost (Ontario Ministry of Health 1976). Ontario's auditor general identified the same problem in 2005 (Office of the Auditor 2005). Then, as now, not only was the price of an LMS unit negotiated, but the units assigned to a particular test were negotiated as well.

Whatever the other benefits for the private laboratories, the LMS unit system created another structural barrier between the community and the hospitals. Hospitals used Dominion Bureau of Statistics units, now the Management Information System (MIS). The MIS relies on a measurement of time taken for each test and is the most widely used system in laboratories in Canada. That these two different workload measurement systems are used comes up again and again as one of the reasons why no reliable cost comparisons can be made between for-profit and hospital laboratories. The lack of reliable data showing that hospitals provide the same service for less is a key argument used by supporters of for-profit laboratories to oppose shifting community work to the hospitals.

Profitable but Not Efficient

As well as benefiting private labs by differentiating community laboratory work, the LMS system is biased towards manual tests, which may be part of the reason why for-profit laboratories are often behind hospitals in the use of automation. A 1994 study found that approximately 82 percent of tests performed in hospitals were automated compared to 72 percent in the private laboratory system, even though for-profit laboratories performed more routine tests. This figure underestimates the extent of hospital automation. Up to 10 percent of hospital tests at that time were so esoteric that they were not even represented in the laboratory fee schedule and were unlikely to have been automated (Ontario Ministry of Health 1994b).

Comments by a non-profit community laboratory, the HICL, to the Task Force on Laboratory Services in 1983, outline how this bias against automation in the for-profit sector works:

> For example, when cholesterol and triglycerides are ordered in a hospital setting, these tests can be performed on an automated chemical analyzer. However a private laboratory could run these two tests on an analyzer without simultaneously functioning channels and invoice the Ontario Health Insurance Plan for L055 — cholesterol at 14 units and L243 — triglycerides at 21 units, for a total bill of 35 LMS units [instead of the 18 maximum if they had used a more sophisticated procedure].[5]

There continue to be strong indications that the private sector does not take advantage of cheaper automated procedures, preferring instead to be less efficient and more profitable. The *Globe and Mail* reported in 2010 that the higher cost for vitamin D tests done in for-profit laboratories is partly due to the fact that they use less automated procedures than are used in the hospitals (Mittelstaedt 2010).

Licensing the Laboratory Sector

In an attempt to curb fraud, over utilization and questionable quality in the private laboratories, in the 1970s the Ontario government enacted a series of regulations. Central among these was the licensing of laboratories and specimen collection centres (SCCs). Licensing medical laboratories had been on and off Ontario's agenda since 1943. Rising costs and quality concerns related to the rapid increase in the number of private laboratories during the 1960s gave the issue increased urgency. A 1969 report on the private laboratories said: "Indeed it has only been in the last few years, with the increase in private laboratory medicine, that there has been a need for legislation of this kind" (Chemical Engineering Research 1969).

Licensing of the laboratory sector was initially done through an amendment to the *Public Health Act*, which came into force on November 1, 1972. In 1984 this part of the act and related amendments were consolidated into the *Laboratory and Specimen Collection Centre Licensing Act*, which is still the primary legislation governing the sector. To encourage cooperation with the licensing program, only licensed laboratories were allowed to bill OHIP for technical laboratory services.

By the end of September 1973, 510 laboratories had been licensed in Ontario (214 in hospitals and 296 privately owned). There had also been a rash of requests for new licences, and the government felt it needed to do more to stop the growth of the sector.

No New Laboratories

On November 15, 1973, the Ontario Cabinet approved changes to the criteria governing licensure designed to improve its ability to limit new laboratories and SCCs. "Public need" was replaced by "public interest." The new rules mandated that "the utilization of existing laboratories and their capacity to handle increased volume" and "the availability of funds" had to be considered in the evaluation of new requests. Cabinet also agreed that, "as a matter of government policy, no new private laboratories should be licensed"; this provision was not to be made public.[6]

Since approval of this policy, all requests for new labs have been met with a polite letter from the director of laboratory services stating that there were already too many labs and only under exceptional circumstances would they be opening new laboratories. In fact no new laboratories have been opened in Ontario since Cabinet took that position.[7] This rule marked the start of a thirty-year history of Conservative governments enacting policy to limit competition in the commercial laboratory sector, which has had the effect of enhancing the profitability and stability of a decreasing number of ever-larger corporations.

The major chains did not challenge the restrictions on opening new laboratories. They were moving in the other direction: buying up smaller operations to increase their market share. They were now anxious to close smaller labs. What they really wanted was more SCCs to collect patient samples, which could be processed in their larger, more centralized facilities. To achieve this goal, they applied pressure on the government to allow the conversion of laboratories into SCCs, effectively circumventing the prohibition on new SCCs.[8] This proposal also had the support of the licensing program: fewer laboratories meant fewer locations to track. Table 2.2 shows that while the number of labs has continued to fall the number of specimen collection centres has increased. Being able to change laboratories into SCCs was only a partial victory for the commercial sector. They were still limited in where they could open new SCCs: a restriction they would challenge when they were a bit bigger, better organized and in need of more business.

Table 2-2   Ontario Laboratories and SCCs, 1967–2008

Year	Hospital	Commercial	Public Health	SCCs
1967	222	112		N/A
1974	227	288	13	188
1993	216	159	13	273
2008	175	32	12	420

Sources: Reports prepared by the Laboratories Branch of the Ministry of Health; Ontario Ministry of Health 1993e, QMP–LS 2008 Review of Activities except the SCC numbers, which come from the Licensing and X-ray Inspection Branch, Ministry of Health. Note: Does not include unlicensed SCCs operating in doctors' offices.

Most commercial laboratories benefited from the restriction on opening new laboratories. The limited market entry increased the value of the smaller laboratories, making it lucrative for them to sell, and the big ones wanted the market share, making it worthwhile for them to buy. The government also used licensing to address quality problems, which added to the pressure on the small laboratories.

Quality Assurance Monitoring

In 1969, the Committee on Healing Arts found that, "it is apparent that there is room for and a need for improvement [in the quality of private laboratories]" (Chemical Engineering Research 1969: 43). When licensing was introduced in 1973 laboratories had to agree to participate in quality assurance programs as a condition of being granted a licence. The Ontario Medical Association (OMA) was given the contract to run the external quality control program, initially called the Laboratory Proficiency Testing Program (LPTP) and changed in 2000 to the Quality Management Program – Laboratory Services (QMP–LS).

While the government was aware of the conflict inherent in having the OMA police its own members, the Ministry of Health dismissed this hazard as no greater a risk than using an outside agency; "in fact, it is probably lower because of the desire of the O.M.A. to protect its reputation."[9] The result was that the profession gained control of another aspect of the laboratory industry, with the reputation of doctors being used to bolster that of the commercial companies.

It was intended that the laboratory quality control program be self-financing. All laboratories, regardless of size, were required to pay the same fee (Ontario Ministry of Health 1974), a system that favoured larger laboratories. However, the program has never paid for itself; with the Ontario government paying the OMA $3.7 million in 2003–04 to run the program (Office of the Auditor 2005). More importantly, the new reporting requirements, forms, education programs and remedial action, while useful in terms of improving quality, had the effect of making it harder for small operators to survive.[10] Even MDS noted that, "the retention of laboratory staff and facilities and participation in the LPTP has become a major problem."[11]

Conflicts of Interest and Overuse

Darlene Berger (1999), in her series of articles on the history of clinical laboratories, identifies the period after 1970 as one of "Fraud and Abuse." While her history deals mostly with the U.S. experience, Canadian corporations have much the same reputation as their U.S. counterparts. Even though convictions for fraud, such as charging the public system for tests that were not done, are rare in Canada, allegations of abuse are common.

In a fee-for-service payment system, a core objective of corporate efforts is to collect and process increasing numbers of samples. Convincing a doctor, often with some form of incentive, to let the laboratory take and process all of that physician's tests is an excellent way of increasing market share and income.

Not only is the lab paid a fee for every test it processes but if it also collects the sample it can bill for labelling the sample and processing the patient, which can be the largest single source of income for a company.

Private laboratory owners aggressively enticed physicians to direct their work to their labs. The simplest of these approaches was the kind proposed by Labcare in 1973 and then MDS in 1982: the lab supplies a phlebotomist to take blood in a doctor's office as long as all the samples go to that laboratory. Other incentives to capture market share included free financial consulting (Plant 1977b), low cost or free equipment such as photocopiers, and subsidized rent. For instance, a laboratory would lease six thousand feet in a building owned by physicians but only occupy one thousand, allowing the physicians to use the other five thousand at little or no cost (Walkom 1994). Or a laboratory would pay $120 per square foot rent while physician tenants would pay $20, if the physicians directed their work to the landlord lab.[12] To further boost business, labs set up programs to pick up samples in private homes and nursing homes for free. Other arrangements were less subtle. The *Toronto Star* told the story of a Toronto lab paying up to $3000 to doctors to direct patients their way (Walkom 1994). Besides offering tangible incentives, pushers of for-profit laboratories appealed to doctors' concerns about cash-strapped hospitals performing community laboratory tests without compensation. One argued: "Surely it will help [the hospital] if we take our work to a private laboratory which can receive appropriate payments for the work we give them."[13]

It was reported in 1996 that roughly one hundred doctors were being investigated for taking kickbacks (Priest 1996; Cohen 1996). Regulation 682 under the *Laboratory and Specimen Centre Collection Act*, passed in 1996, placed tighter restrictions on the benefits laboratories could confer on physicians who order laboratory tests. One section specifically prohibits beneficial rental agreements, though it exempts any lease in effect on the date the amendment passed. In 1998, John Nicol and Stephanie Nolen interviewed nine doctors for an article in *Maclean's Magazine,* "all of whom confirmed that the practices continue" despite the new regulations.

A 1999 agreement between Gamma-Dynacare and YFMC Health Care/ Med-Emerg International, a for-profit company that manages medical clinics, contained kickbacks of 6 percent of net OHIP billings as a "contribution for the cost of collecting specimens" and 15 percent for non-insured samples, paid by Gamma-Dynacare to YFMC.[14] This agreement continues a history of private labs paying financial incentives to increase volume, but takes it one step further. The for-profit medical clinic management firm, YFMC, has an incentive to pressure doctors and patients in their clinics to order more tests and, to realize even greater profits, to order more uninsured tests.

Regulatory Attempts to Control Overuse

In an attempt to reduce overuse and control costs, the government focused on policies aimed at individual doctors. Treating physicians as the source of the overuse problem had the support of MDS, whose president argued: "To me the important thing is the ordering pattern of the physicians in the community where the patient originates."[15]

Initially, firm limits were placed on the tests that could be done by physicians in their offices and strict rules were imposed regulating who could perform them. Predictably, the consequences of these policies were not in the public interest. As in the 1960s, when remuneration for many tests done in a doctor's office ended, there was no incentive in a fee-for-service regime for doctors to perform the tests. Why not reduce their workload and send the patient to a laboratory, increasingly a private one, for the test? If the doctor also owned part of the lab, the increased income was bonus. These regulations resulted in more tests for commercial laboratories and underlined the potential conflict of interest between doctors and commercial laboratories.

In 1971, Alan Lawrence, minister of health, raised conflict-of-interest concerns at an OMA convention: "Why do you [the medical profession] permit physicians to have an interest in laboratories, and why does significantly greater use (and cost) of laboratory services arise in circumstances where physicians have a financial interest in the laboratories being used?"[16]

The issue of conflict of interest came back on the public agenda in 1977 when charges were laid against doctor-owned ABKO Laboratories for defrauding the Ministry of $500,000 (*Globe and Mail* 1977a). The jailing of an NDP MPP for refusing to reveal a source of information on laboratory corruption also highlighted the issue (*Globe and Mail* 1977c). The government responded in September 1977 by enacting regulation O.R. 195/77 under the *Public Health Act* to prevent, "legally qualified medical practitioners from being owners of laboratories or... having any interest therein."[17]

The OMA opposed the regulation as "unnecessary, discriminatory and foster[ing] commercial laboratory ownership" (*Globe and Mail* 1977b: 5). As noted earlier, the profession has always argued that ownership by doctors, particularly laboratory specialists, was essential for quality. The assumption was that doctors would only order tests that were needed by their patients and any unscrupulous doctors would be dealt with by the College of Physicians and Surgeons of Ontario regulations on malpractice.[18] The regulation was first postponed while it went through a series of backroom negotiations with the medical profession and was finally repealed in 1979. Instead, the *Health Discipline Act* regulations were amended so that physicians would be liable to charges of professional misconduct if they were shown to have an interest in a diagnostic facility from which they ordered medically unnecessary tests (Ontario Ministry of Health 1978). No concerns were raised about the possibility that medically unnecessary tests might be sent to an arms-length company. This amendment kept the policing of the profession under the profession's control so was not opposed by the OMA.

It seems likely that physicians having direct ownership of a company from which they ordered laboratory tests did increase use but it was fast becoming irrelevant. By 1977, only sixteen of 244 private labs had a physician who or-dered tests as a direct owner. Sixty-six more labs had physician owners, mostly pathologists, who did not see patients so did not order tests. The rest were non-physician owned and 89 percent of corporate-owned laboratories were held by shareholders whose identities could not be discerned by the Ministry (Gold, Plant and MacKillop 1979). MDS, for example, traded on the Toronto and Montreal Stock Exchanges, and, as they informed the Ministry, "We have no idea whether qualified medical practitioners hold shares in MDS, either directly or indirectly, that conceivably might have an interest conflict because they refer patients to our laboratories."[19]

The problem was shifting from one of individual conflict of interest to a societal one. Dispersed shareholding in private health care corporations ties the welfare of those who depend upon dividend income to the increased use of those corporations in the delivery of public health care. The case of LifeLabs, the purchaser of MDS, illustrates the problem most clearly. LifeLabs is owned by the pension plan of some public sector laboratory workers: for a good pension they require that a company that will take away their jobs and hurt their access to affordable and accessible healthcare make a profit.

Challenging Licensing Restrictions
After the introduction of licensing, there were attempts by physicians, either in conjunction with commercial enterprises or by themselves, to circumvent the new restrictions. Labcare Services offered to provide a technician for in-office phlebotomy, effectively establishing an unlicensed SCC, and handle the physi-cian's billing in exchange for a contract to process all that physician's laboratory work.[20] This company was immediately reported to the government and the OMA by other commercial laboratories, including both MDS and Kipling Laboratories,[21] and the arrangement was stopped.

After aggressively moving to limit completion in the early 1970s, by 1979 MDS and the other large chains increased pressure on the Ministry to allow them to establish new SCCs in more lucrative markets, often close to hospitals and doctors' buildings. In November 1982, MDS engaged in a form of civil disobedi-ence by entering into an agreement with a physicians' office in Elmira to sup-ply a technician to take samples in the office and pay the physicians a monthly fee: that is, they established an unlicensed SCC.[22] The physicians at the office received a free worker, income and good access for their patients. MDS cornered the market on these physicians' patients. The other benefit to the physicians was, since the lab specimens were taken in their office, they were able to bill OHIP for the venipuncture and then MDS was able to bill again for processing the sample. This arrangement was very similar to the one that Labcare tried to establish in 1973, the one that MDS helped stop.

Ministry briefing notes in 1985 on how to handle questions from Peter Moon, a *Globe and Mail* investigative reporter writing on corruption in the laboratory industry, reveal official concerns about double billing and collaboration between doctors and labs to circumvent the restriction on new SCCs. These notes also show the support given by the OMA to doctors and large private laboratory corporations to challenge government policy.

> [The] apparent duplication of payment [was] brought to the attention of OHIP personnel [by the Laboratory Branch of the MOH]…. The OMA Central Tariff Committee's response was that the present payment protocol should remain unchanged but offered no reason for their position. The combined effect of the legislative exemption for physicians [being paid for and performing tests] and the present OHIP payment structure for specimen collection services encourages collaboration between private laboratories and physicians in establishing unlicensed SCCs.[23]

MDS was charged with opening an unlicensed SCC in Elmira and an unlicensed SCC in Sault Saint Marie, "essentially across the street from two hospitals."[24] Six other charges against laboratories, including Bramalea Medical Holdings, Cybermedix and Donway Diagnostics, were laid about the same time. MDS was found guilty at two lower courts on the Elmira charges before having the conviction overturned by the Ontario Court of Appeal. The higher court found that since the SCC was in a doctors' office, the doctors controlled the specimen collection and so it was permitted under regulations that allowed venipuncture in doctors' offices. After the court ruling in favour of MDS, licensing control of SCCs became "illusory."[25] Community laboratory costs continued to increase significantly above most other health care costs. It was estimated that in 1995 there were 250 unlicensed SCCs in doctors' offices (Gamble 2002).

In 2010 there were 420 licensed SCCs in Ontario. While the Ministry maintains that it controls the location of the centres according to public interest criteria (Tse 2010, personal communication), the inclusion of a clause in the 2006 agreement with the OAML requiring the private labs to consult with the Ministry before moving an SCC indicates there are still some problems in this area. Requests to the Ministry to identify these problems were met with silence.

There is nothing illegal about these companies going to court to challenge laws they think are unfair: nor should there be. The difficulty arises when these for-profit companies provide medically essential services. Rather than working to improve access, quality and efficiency of the public system, these corporations use their money and connections to expand their market share, which means increasing their share of public health care dollars. Thus, they undermine nonprofit delivery, both financially and institutionally, for private gain.

The other tension created by allowing private corporations to deliver an essential service is that reasonable public goals, such as improving access for patients, controlling abuse, and the efficient delivery of services, which providing a coordinated system of collection centres could do, are more difficult to achieve when these companies are also advocating for more centres to increase their volumes and incomes. This conflict would not exist if essential services were delivered not for private profit but solely for the benefit of communities.

Positive Cost Containment Programs

The government and the OMA, as part of their efforts to control costs, introduced programs to help individual doctors order only necessary tests. In 1977, the government tried to decrease the number of tests by changing the laboratory requisition form from an open ended document to a list of tests so that doctors would be forced to identify the specific tests they wanted. This approach did have a short-term effect, but a year later the level of test ordering in the community had surpassed previous highs and continued to grow faster on a per capita basis than in the hospitals. This phenomenon, utilization rates returning to pre-intervention levels, is common when new programs are introduced in fee-for-service environments (Bunting and van Walraven 2003). In 1990s, when hard caps took away the incentive to increase volumes, two programs to improve physician ordering, one through individual education (Bunting and van Walraven 2003) and one through improving requisition forms and guidelines (van Walraven, Vivek and Chan 1998) had more successful long-term results. The fact that the number of laboratory tests in the community did not decrease until government funding to the laboratory corporations was capped in 1993 indicates that the primary source of the problem was not family doctors but the funding structure and the profit motive.

Focusing on individual doctors as the cause of the overuse problem is the corollary of biomedicine's focus on physicians as the arbiters of good health care and the system's gatekeepers. Both of these aspects of biomedicine are rooted in capitalist ideology, which focuses on the individual rather than systemic problems. When something goes wrong, it is assumed to be a problem with an individual physician's practice, with the result that other factors causing an increase in the volume of laboratory services are given little attention or ignored all together, e.g., the usefulness of new tests, the profit motive of the commercial laboratories, the increasing number of health care providers, fee-for-service payment mechanisms, the lack of system integration and the underfunding of hospitals. Downplaying these concerns makes it more likely that for-profit laboratories and private capital accumulation will be favoured when new policies are introduced.

The for-profit initiatives, schemes and arrangements that have been discussed are all directed at boosting market share and the volume of laboratory business, all of which involve a cost to the system. Since the primary payer in Canada is public health insurance, they all lead to increases in public spending on health care and thus undermine the sustainability of our public system.

Consolidation of the Laboratory Industry

Government interventions aimed at controlling costs — licensing and conflict-of-interest regulations — were not very effective at achieving that goal, but they did play a significant role in the supporting the corporatization, consolidation and expansion of for-profit laboratory corporations. In 1966, 90 percent of private laboratories were owned by physicians, the remaining 10 percent were owned by "chemists, technicians, non-profit-making groups and municipalities" (Chemical Engineering Research 1969: 7). Most laboratories were sole proprietorships, but corporate chains were starting to emerge. The largest of these was Pathologists' Services, with sixteen laboratories in Toronto, which was run a bit like a franchise operation: individual labs were owned by pathologists under the "supervision" of three pathologists, two of whom were on staff at Toronto's Doctors' Hospital. They all used similar procedures: training and staff were interchangeable. "A percentage of each analysis fee is given to Pathologists' Services in payment for supplies and for professional assistance" (Chemical Engineering Research 1969: 13).

After 1968, a number of forces led to rapid changes in the laboratory landscape. Assured payment for laboratory tests, a potentially ever-expanding fee-for-service market and no controls on the ownership of labs quickly attracted the interest of private capital. At the same time, automation increased the need for capital investment.

The push from the private sector to expand the use of laboratory services and to tie pathologists into private sector growth is evidenced in a 1970 prospectus from Cybermedix, "seeking capital for expansion."[26] Cybermedix was inviting doctors to be involved in "the glamour and excitement of a 'growth industry,'" the health care industry. One of its corporate objectives was, "to maintain and operate a series of fully automated testing laboratories throughout Canada and the United States."

By 1983, five companies received 51 percent of all community laboratory payments, with over half of that going to MDS.[27] The commercial laboratories were now providing 38 percent (1982) of all provincial laboratory services (Ontario Council, 1982), up from 8 percent in 1967 (Chemical 1969). In 2007, three multinationals controlled 93 percent of Ontario's community laboratory

Table 2-3 Consolidation of Ontario's For-Profit Laboratory Industry

Year	For-Profit Laboratory Companies	Labs	Percent Incorporated	Percent Community Work to Top Three For-Profit Companies
1967	83	112	33	
1975	126	253		30.5
1993	62	159		
2005	11	49	100	93

Sources: Chemical Engineering Research 1969, Plant 1977b, Ontario Ministry of Health 1993a, Laboratories Branch, Ontario Ministry of Health and Long Term Care.

services and performed approximately 50 percent of all the laboratory tests in Ontario.

Ontario Association of Medical Laboratories

While the government and the OMA were engaged in battle over what should be done about doctors' overuse of laboratory services, the for-profit corporations were expanding and becoming a political force. In 1976, the commercial laboratories formed the Ontario Association of Medical Laboratories (OAML), an industry association controlled by the larger laboratories. Voting was originally allocated on the percentage of market share; currently the board consists of two representatives from each of the three large laboratories and one for all the small labs (Sutherland 2007).

The creation of the OAML allowed the for-profit laboratory industry a formal presence in government decision-making. While no specific government policy mandated that the OAML or private laboratories have representation on government committees, the OAML lobbied for and was granted, "an equal voice with other sectors" on the Laboratory Advisory Committees, committees set up to advise district health councils, and the Provincial Laboratory Advisory Committee (Plant 1977a). The OAML became a partner with the OMA in setting LMS units and prices for laboratory tests.

The OAML's role, like any industry lobby group, was to protect the interests of its members. In this instance, the job includes working to weaken the public sector. Briefing notes for the minister of health in 1977 (Plant 1977a) and again in 1985[28] report that the main concerns brought by the OAML to the Ministry involved reducing the role of hospitals and the non-profit Hospitals In-Common Laboratory (HICL) in community laboratory services

Even when the for-profit sector was small, it used its influence to reduce the role of public, non-profit laboratory services. Starting in 1969, paid consultants to for-profit laboratories tried to stop the formation of the HICL, and opposition from the OMA pathology section caused the Ontario Hospital Services Commission to delay the HICL's expansion into new facilities (Freedman 1970). In addition, a campaign of misinformation run by the private laboratories tried to undercut a hospital-based community laboratory program in Hamilton.[29]

A key component of the for-profit sector's attack on hospitals was the demand for incontrovertible data that hospitals could do a better job of providing laboratory services to community patients. The lack of hard data was cited many times as a reason for more study and less action. On a funding proposal to allow the Hamilton hospitals to do more community work, the acting director of the Licensing Branch commented: "One can be relatively certain, if these questions [about the quality of data] are not addressed now, the Ontario Association of Medical Laboratories, for their own partisan reasons and in self defence [will object]."[30] In 1982, the quality of the data and the difficulty of comparing hospital and community data were used to undercut the Hospital Outpatient Pilot Project, the largest project to encourage hospitals to perform more community work.

As well as demanding hard data, the OAML was instrumental in ensuring that these data could not be obtained. Gathering comparative data was made extremely difficult, if not impossible, by the different payment and workload measuring systems engineered by doctors and the private sector.

Staff Conflict of Interest

The presence of the OAML on official committees was not the only avenue of influence of the private labs in government decision-making. In 1977, the provincial director of laboratory services noted that, "MDS enjoys a considerable degree of influence with the medical profession... which translates into having an indirect, but nonetheless effective, voice relating to the annual revisions in the LMS unit assignments" (Plant 1977b: 4). The first executive director of the OAML, Dr. Sawyer, was a past president of the OMA. The interconnections were fluid and they worked against hospital laboratories and in favour of the commercial sector.

The more serious conflict of interest was between the doctors, usually pathologists, who were both medical directors of for-profit laboratories and staff doctors running hospital laboratories. The 1982 Task Force on Laboratory Services found that, "of the 171 physicians in private laboratories, at least 156 also hold single or multiple hospital appointments" (Ontario Council of Health 1982: 112). This fact could partially explain why hospitals did not always go out of their way to attract more community work. In 1995, forty-seven hospital laboratories shared a medical director with a for-profit laboratory.[31] The problem came to a head in Sudbury in 1996 when the medical director of the Sudbury General Hospital, who was also a director of an MDS laboratory, attempted to transfer most of the hospital's laboratory work to MDS. Opposition from local health professionals and the community thwarted this plan (St. Pierre 1996).

In 2007, eighteen hospitals still shared a laboratory director with a commercial laboratory; nine of these were smaller northern hospitals and four were Niagara region hospitals[32]: both are areas with long histories of private laboratories performing a variety of work for public hospitals.

Political Conflict of Interest — Money and Personnel

Strong personal connections were established between the private laboratories and government in the 1990s, a time crucial to cementing the political and economic position of the private laboratories. Just as the NDP was forming government in Ontario in 1990, MDS enticed former NDP provincial secretary Brian Harling to join their organization to take charge of community and political relations, not just in Ontario but across Canada. MDS also hired former NDP cabinet ministers in British Columbia and Saskatchewan, as well as officials attached to the Liberals, to work on their behalf.

The Latner family, principals in Gamma-Dynacare, established a presence in Mike Harris's Progressive Conservative government through their close friend Tom Long, who was Harris's chief of staff and managed his 1995 and 1997 election campaigns. Early in Harris's first term, the Latner family received a number of beneficial rulings, including one that opened up home care services to competition, which provided a market for their home care company, Comcare, and another that closed competition in the laboratory market to protect their interests in Gamma-Dynacare.

Other provinces have also had a significant crossovers of personnel that have created potential conflict-of-interest situations. For example, Jennifer Rice, a former medical director of DynaLIFE, headed Alberta's laboratory transition team, which recommended DynaLIFE as one of the two laboratories to provide a centralized cytology service (Lang 2009). In British Columbia, the former president and CEO of the Vancouver Coastal Health Authority became CEO of LifeLabs, its main competitor for community laboratory work. A former president of MDS, Alan Torrie, had also been CEO of Joseph Brant Hospital in Burlington, Ontario (Fuller 1998).

Personal ties between governments and the laboratories are supported by financial ties. For-profit laboratories continue to be among the top financial backers of Ontario's Liberals and Conservatives. In 2007, an Ontario election year, for-profit laboratories donated $55,975 to the two parties, and in 2008 they gave $33,625. These amounts underestimate the level of financial support because they are only the donations to the central party office from the corporations; no personal donations or donations to individual riding associations are included.

It is worth noting that hospitals and public health labs are not allowed to make political donations or publicly support a political party. There are also strong implicit prohibitions on the level and type of criticisms they can make of their political masters. These restrictions are another dimension of the uneven playing field that disadvantages collective solutions to social problems.

Summary

In 1970, most politicians, bureaucrats and health policy analysts felt that private laboratory corporations were a serious problem, yet by 1990 they were providing 45 percent of Ontario's publicly funded laboratory services and were becoming the major laboratory force, both economically and politically. Despite twenty years of clear political goals to decrease laboratory use and increase integration of the laboratory system, costs continued to rise and the barriers between different laboratory sectors were firmer.

While the NDP and the Ontario Public Service Employees Union had called for an end to funding the for-profit laboratory corporations, there was little appetite for this type of anti-market solution in Conservative and Liberal governments and no broad campaign to stop private delivery of publicly funded health care services. Rather, it was felt that concerns about the private corporations could be satisfied by licensing the sector, controlling conflicts of interest and improving quality. These measures did not work. Biomedicine and the pro-market bias in the Ontario government turned each of these potentially socially beneficial interventions into factors supporting the consolidation and growth of ever-larger laboratory companies and undercutting the public provision of laboratory services.

Attempts to increase the public provision of services are the focus of the next chapter, and these were moderately successful. But the rising power of the for-profit providers and the impact on Ontario politics of a shift in the structure of the global economy to favour private corporations limited their success. By 1990, the private laboratory sector was on the verge of consolidating its political power, which is the story in Chapter Four.

Notes

1. "Cost Control of Medical Laboratories," May 17, 1972. AO, RG 10-6-0, B254828.
2. "Bulk Billings for Hospital Out-Patient Radiology," February 5, 1974. AO, RG 10-18, barcode 112932, box 2, file 7-47/75(H).
3. Minutes of the MOH Policy Committee, March 4, 1975. AO, RG 10-45, barcode 258888, box 3.
4. "Minister's Meeting, October 1, 1974," AO, RG 10-18, barcode 112932, file: 9-128173.
5. "Re: the report of the Task Force on Laboratory Services 1982," HICL's letter of January 31, 1984, to the Chairman of Ontario Council of Health. AO, RG 10-247, container 8, acc.28303, B212503.
6. Ontario Cabinet Meeting of November 15, 1973, Minute no: 3/63/73. AO, RG 10-18, barcode 112932, box 2.
7. "Consolidation of Private Laboratory Operations by Conversions to Specimen Collection Centers: Brief," October 19, 1976. AO, RG 10-18, box 15, B156793.
8. Ibid.
9. "Continuation of the O.M.A. as the Agency Appointed by the Ministry of Health, to Conduct Proficiency Testing in all Medical Laboratories in Ontario," undated MOH report. AO, RG10 – 18, barcode 112932, Box 2, file 0-128173.
10. "Laboratory Proficiency Testing Program Annual Report – May 1979." AO.
11. "Consolidation of Private Laboratory Operations by Conversions to Specimen Collection Centers," op. cit.
12. Bruce Thomson, a pathologist in Georgetown, letter to I. Jadusingh, Medical Laboratory Consultants in Calgary, May 12, 1997; and "Ministerial Information Book," AO, RG 10-39, box5, B383120, file: info book.
13. E.G. Warburton, "Presentation to Provincial Laboratory Advisory Committee, Thursday, June 29, 1978," August 11, 1978. AO. RG10-39, file:MB202.
14. Ivan Flaschner, Vice President, Corporate Affairs, Gamma Dynacare, letter to Don Wilson, YFMC/Med-Emerg International, November 8, 1999.
15. Wilfred G. Lewitt, President, MDS Health Group Limited, letter to S.W. Martin, Deputy Minister, Department of Health, July 20, 1973. AO.
16. "Partnership in Progress," remarks by the Honourable A.B.R. Lawrence, Minister of Health, to the Ontario Medical Association, Friday May 14, 1971. AO RG 10-6-0, B254828.
17. "Background Regarding the Ownership of Medical Laboratories by Legally Qualified Medical Practitioners," briefing document attached to memo from Dennis Timbrell, Minister of Health, to W.A. Backley, December 9, 1977. AO.
18. Ibid.
19. D.M. Phillips, Vice President of MDS Laboratories, letter to D. Corder, Director,

Laboratory and Specimen Collection Centres, June 3, 1977. AO, RG 10-39, file:0 legislation SG.10.01.

20. Letter from A.R. Adams, President, Kipling Medical Laboratories, to H. Sharpe, Director of Laboratory Licenses, October 25, 1973. AO, RG 10-39, file: Laboratory Tests-Labcare services 1974.

21. "Ontario Regulation 463/73 – Laboratory Tests Performed by Qualified Medical Practitioners," February 12, 1974. AO, RG 10-39, file: Laboratory Tests-Labcare services 1974.

22. "Synopsis of Review of Laboratory Utilization and Referral Patterns Regarding Application to Establish New Specimen Collection Center: MDS Health Group Limited, 4 Park Avenue West, Elmira," August 15, 1983. AO RG 10-39, box 5, B383120.

23. "*Globe and Mail* Request for Interview on Private laboratories," Ministry of Health, May 8, 1984. AO, RG 10-39, box 5, b383120.

24. "Ministers Briefing Book: Laboratory Services Branch," May 21, 1985, p. 94. AO, RG-39, box 5, B383120.

25. Ibid.

26. "Cybermedix Limited," prospectus from gordon, eberts and company limited [name not capitalized]. Attached to a letter from M.O. Klotz, Chief Pathologist at the Ottawa Civic Hospital, to J.D. Galloway, Medical Director, St Joseph's Hospital Hamilton, April 10, 1970. AO.

27. "Minster's Briefing Book: Laboratory Services Branch," May 21, 1985, p. 22. AO, RG-39, box 5, B383120.

28. "Assistant Deputy Minister's Briefing Book: Ontario Association of Medical Laboratories (OAML)," May 21, 1985. AO, RG 10-39, box 5, B3833120.

29. "Report on the meeting of the Task Force on Laboratory Services, Ontario Council of Health, November 30, 1981," AO, RG 10-247, container 1, Acc 28303, B212530.

30. "Hamilton Laboratory Funding Proposal," April 5, 1978. AO, RG 10-39, file:57.01.01.

31. List of Laboratory Medical Directors released under Freedom of Information request file number 95502-MOH on January 16, 1996.

32. "Laboratory Director List," the Laboratories Branch of the MOH, March, 2007.

Chapter 3

Support for Non-Profit Delivery

For-profit laboratory corporations thrived in the 1970s and 1980s in spite of a general institutional distrust of them and government policies designed to control them. The most significant challenges to the for-profit laboratories came from programs using hospital laboratories to analyze specimens from community patients. The impetus for these programs often came from the public hospitals, with support and encouragement from the Ministry. Hospitals used their organizational resources to improve their inpatient services and reach out into the community. This institutional base, the result of a half century of progressive struggle, provided a challenge to the expansion of the for-profit industry.

Hospital Regionalization Initiatives

With the increase in hospital costs in Ontario from $162 million in 1959 to $573 million in 1968, a 250 percent increase,[1] the Ontario Hospital Services Commission (OHSC), the government body responsible for administering Ontario's hospitals, supported programs to integrate hospital services and control costs. Laboratory services was one area where both cost control and integration were considered achievable.

The expansion of the scientific basis of medicine, the increasing volume of tests and changes in technology (e.g., the introduction of high cost equipment that could either analyze multiple samples at once or perform several tests on one sample simultaneously or both) gave further impetus to hospitals to coordinate their laboratory resources. Trends in the United States towards regional and centralized laboratory structures helped shape these initiatives (Jentz 1968).

In 1967, Ottawa started to centralize laboratory services with extra funding from the Ministry of Health.[2] In March 1972, an inter-hospital laboratory services program in Huron and Perth Counties brought together hospitals in Clinton, Exeter, Goderich, Listowel, Palmerston, St. Mary's, Seaforth, Stratford and Wingham.[3] Kingston began to regionalize its services, eventually developing the Clinical Laboratories of Eastern Ontario, a network that services the small, nearby hospitals using Kingston General Hospital's expertise and more comprehensive capabilities (More, Sengupta and Manley 2000). Cochrane developed a district laboratory service in which "7 or 8 hospitals send everything to one laboratory."[4] Hospitals in Kenora and Rainy River Districts developed a coordination program to share technologists (Ontario Ministry of Health 1979). Sudbury[5] and St. Catherines[6] were also working on coordination of local services.

Many of the initiatives started in the 1960s and 1970s developed into long-term cooperation on inpatient programs but were less successful at integrating hospital and community work. Two of the most successful hospital initiatives that did involve processing community specimens were the Hospitals In-Common Laboratory (HICL)[7] based in Toronto and the Hamilton Health Sciences Laboratory Program (HHSLP).[8]

Hospitals In-Common Laboratory

The HICL started as a project between Toronto General Hospital and Mount Sinai Hospital; the Ottawa Civic Hospital was originally involved as well, but soon decided to withdraw and concentrate on its own regional project. The HICL was designed to pool some of the hospitals' lower volume inpatient tests so that they would have enough volume in one place to justify buying the newest technology (Freeman 1970). Alan Pollard, a clinical biochemist and one of the participants in the formation of the HICL, described it as an "environment of innovation" in which pathologists, clinical chemists, administrators and other hospital staff came together to experiment with ways to make hospital laboratory services more effective and efficient (Pollard 1975). In 1968, the first test was performed at the new joint laboratory, for the common blood chemical urea.

The project was developed through a series of meetings open to anyone with an interest, similar to a classic community development process and serving a similar purpose. The project developed a broad base of support, which protected it from the opposition of for-profit laboratories and parochial hospital interests. When physicians linked to private laboratories supported a motion at one of the pivotal organizing meetings to stop the initiative the motion was defeated. The OMA's pathology section raised a "hue and cry" about the HICL from 1969 to 1971.[9] They expressed concern that the HICL would become an "irreversible" monolith "unresponsive to local community health needs and to the requirements of good patient care."[10] But their real concern was the possibility that laboratory services might develop outside of pathologists' control and compete with the for-profit labs that were making some pathologists rich.

These conflicts within the medical community over the HICL illustrate a central tension in biomedicine, the conflict between individualism and professional medical service. On the one hand, non-profit hospitals provide specialists with an environment in which to practise medicine to its full scope and maintain significant control over their practices, activities limited by for- profit laboratories as they became larger. On the other hand, as we have seen, doctors, primarily pathologists, demand their right as autonomous practitioners and arbiters of quality to own laboratories, which played a key role in the development of the for-profits. Nonetheless, some pathologists were central to the development of non-profit alternatives, and they became more unified in their defence of hospital laboratories as the larger commercial laboratories became the only community option.

Government support for the HICL came early. The laboratory was initially funded by special grants from the OHSC, which were funnelled through

Toronto General Hospital.[11] These grants covered operating costs, set-up costs and the purchase of equipment. Channelling the funds through hospitals left them in charge and ensured that the HICL's expenses fell under the *HIDSA* and were therefore shared with the federal government. Key principles of the new organization were that it would augment, not compete with, existing hospital laboratory services, and it would work to increase efficiency, quality and integration in the system.

In 1974, the government stopped directly funding the HICL. If hospitals wanted to continue to use the service, they would have to pay for it out of their global budgets — which hospitals did. The Ministry's Policy and Priority Advisory Committee recognized the HICL's success: "the In-Common Laboratory Program has been very successful in providing a better service at a much lower cost [than the private labs]."[12] And to encourage its continued operation, the government covered the HICL's unexpected deficit of $70,000 in 1974 and gave a one-time increase to the global funding of hospitals that had been using the HICL's services before direct funding was stopped.[13]

The HICL became a self-supporting, non-profit corporation that was separate from the hospitals but maintained good relationships with them. As well as handling some bulk tests for hospitals as the transportation network between hospitals developed, many community hospitals started shipping less common and experimental tests through the HICL to the large teaching hospital laboratories. This service grew from connecting twenty-two hospitals in 1971 to connecting 166 by 1981 (HICL 1981). This became known as "the grid," a service still provided by HICL.

The HICL Moves into the Community

The HICL also provided a structure capable of directing community work to hospital laboratories, which it started to do in 1977. In June 1976, A.D.S. Laboratories in Bramalea went bankrupt, leading to a suspension of their licence to operate a laboratory. The owners of the building that leased space to A.D.S. appealed to their MPP, Premier Bill Davis, for help. Self-described supporters of Davis, they wanted him to hasten the process of obtaining a new laboratory for their building.[14]

The HICL's chair, R.M. McLuckie, wrote to Gary Chatfield, the assistant deputy minister of health, proposing that the HICL collect the outpatient work in the Brampton area and "flow the bulk of the work to the [local] hospital and the remainder through our grid." He argued that this was a situation where, "the HICL could really demonstrate its ability to work as a non-profit laboratory." In a friendly push to "Gary," McLuckie made the case that, "the time has come… when the Ministry must make a decision," and asked that the licence for A.D.S. be transferred to the HICL, which it was.[15]

Having an SCC feed samples to a hospital laboratory was not unique. Other hospitals provided this service. What was unique was that the HICL would receive money from OHIP for each test, as a for-profit laboratory would, and then pay a hospital to process the test. It was agreed that the HICL would only receive a percentage of what the commercial laboratories were paid for the same service. This reduction in payment avoided a direct confrontation with the private labs and provided an opportunity for the non-profit hospital-based structure to prove its worth.

In 1977, the HICL started billing OHIP at 30 cents per LMS unit, 84.5 percent of the fee usually paid to the private labs. This per unit rate was not changed until 1984, when it rose to 32 cents per LMS unit, or 71% percent of the rate then paid to the for-profit laboratories.[16] During that time, the LMS for-profits' unit rate had risen from 35.5 cents to 46.3 cents, a 30 percent increase. In 1986, the rate for the HICL was renegotiated to 75 percent of the fee paid to the commercial labs (Ontario Ministry of Health 1993a).

The HICL's billing practices were also different from the for-profits', though this time the difference worked in its favour. It was allowed to bulk bill OHIP for its services rather than billing for each individual test. It had to keep the same documentation as the other laboratories for auditing purposes, but bulk billing resulted in decreased clerical costs.[17] Bulk billing indicates a level of trust in the non-profit sphere that did not exist towards the for-profits, and this lack of trust led to higher administrative costs for the government when dealing with for-profit corporations.

A briefing note to the minister of health describes how the Ministry had been "receptive" to the HICL's community outreach and that they were monitoring the HICL's "economic performance closely to ensure that costs do not exceed, and are in fact less than, private laboratory reimbursement levels (Plant 1977a)." In 1981, the provincial coordinator of laboratory services noted that the benefits of the HICL included the following: allowing hospitals to augment their own work increasing "test cost efficiency"; coordination between community laboratory work and inpatient work for both patients and physicians; consultation services for physicians; and a "dependable" laboratory system for hospital administrators. At that time, the HICL was paying "well over $5 million to hospitals for work processed."[18] The case of the HICL shows how an integrated non-profit approach can meet the needs of community patients while decreasing cost and maintaining quality.

Hamilton Health Sciences Laboratory Program

Hamilton developed a program quite different from that of the HICL, which also used hospitals to process community laboratory work. Preliminary work establishing the program began in 1965 under the auspices of hospitals in Hamilton and Burlington. It was coordinated by faculty at McMaster University and through the District Health Council.[19] In 1970, the government purchased capital equipment for the Hamilton initiative and funded it as a five-year pilot project in 1972.[20] The Ministry decided to purchase the equipment outright because it would make it easier to gain federal cost-sharing. In 1973, the program established seven community collection stations, an at-home specimen collection service and collection services for the surrounding rural area and nursing homes: all of which funnelled tests into hospital laboratories (Brain et al. 1976).

In 1977, at the end of the pilot project, intense negotiations took place between the Ministry and the HHSLP. In the new climate of fiscal austerity and increased support for private sector solutions the government did not want to give any money to the HHSLP to provide community laboratory tests. The hospitals responded to governments' budget concerns by arguing that if more funding was not made available, the for-profit sector would end up providing the service at a greater cost. The hospitals won the day, with the Ministry continuing to fund the program, and by 1990, the HHSLP had settled into a stable funding arrangement in which the Ministry provided a small capped yearly increase to meet the additional workload for community services (McQueen and Bailey 1993b).

By 1980, the program was processing roughly 40 percent of the tests ordered by Hamilton's community physicians, "but it was difficult to arrive at a precise figure because there are commercial laboratories in Toronto who have paid personnel working in physicians' offices in Hamilton and other centres to pick up specimens which are then processed in the large Toronto laboratories."[21] In 1990–91, the HHSLP serviced 160,000 community patients and made 21,000 house calls (McQueen and Bailey 1993b).

The HHSLP differed from the HICL in that it was run by a group of hospitals rather than by a separate non-profit corporation that cooperated with hospitals. Second, it was funded primarily from the hospitals' global budgets, with small financial top-ups from the province, compared to the HICL, which received fee-for-service payments that were a percentage of those paid to the for-profit laboratories and then purchased services from hospitals.

The two also had similarities. Both were long-term, stable public sector models that were cheaper to use than commercial laboratories and provided integration of inpatient and community laboratory services. They were both effectively controlled by laboratory specialists within non-profit corporate structures and funded by the state. They are both evidence that the public sector was prepared to develop, and capable of developing, services to meet emerging health care needs. They also indicate that within the broad category of collective responses to social needs, there is a range of options.

Other Hospital-Community Initiatives

Besides the HICL and HHSLP through the 1970s there were numerous other proposals to the MOH for extra funding for hospitals to expand their outpatient services. These other proposals met with less long-term success.

In 1973, Sensenbrenner Hospital in Kapuskasing wanted to take over the operations of Northern Laboratories, a for-profit laboratory, and become the major supplier of laboratory services for Kapuskasing and District. This required additional capital funding and special arrangements for operating costs, but was expected to lead to a decrease in total laboratory costs of $101,000 per year.[22] Hospitals in the Niagara Region, Hanover, Trenton, Mississauga, Peterborough, the Brant Region[23] and Lennox and Addington all submitted proposals to prevent "a shift of hospital laboratory work to the private sector in the community with a resultant savings to the ministry."[24] The Ottawa General Hospital[25] and the Ottawa Civic Hospital [26] both received extra funds to process community specimens from their family practice units.

The increase in hospital requests for more funding for community laboratory work was heavily influenced by funding restrictions put in place as the government tried to control health care costs, a process that culminated in the province's anti-inflation program in 1976. These cuts were exacerbated by the passage of the federal government's *Established Programs Financing Act*, which reduced federal transfers to the provinces for social programs, including health care.

These cuts were the beginning of neoliberal restructuring in Canada. While the emerging political project was to provide more opportunities for private profit under the guise of cost cutting, the spate of proposals from community doctors and hospitals for maintaining and expanding hospital-based community services shows there were viable non-profit alternatives which better meet the objective of a sustainable health care system. These initiatives highlight three points. First, hospitals and other non-profit organizations have seriously considered innovative steps to integrate inpatient and community services. Second, all of these plans proposed providing outpatient services at less cost than the for-profit laboratories. Finally, as evidence of the contradictory forces as work in government and society, the Ministry was often responsive to requests from hospitals to process community laboratory work, though it was not always possible to determine the final official response to some of the individual requests.

Laboratory Outpatient Pilot Project

The pressure from the non-profit sector, as well as the continuing increase in private sector service costs, prompted the government to undertake a coordinated pilot program to expand hospital community services. Under the leadership of Miville Fournier, the recently hired first coordinator of diagnostic services, the Laboratory Services Planning Team, a group of Ministry officials representing the different branches of government concerned with laboratory services, prepared a provincial policy paper on the funding of hospitals for community laboratory services. After multiple submissions, a pilot project gained Cabinet approval and was made operational in Regulation 796/80 on September 19, 1980. The details of the Laboratory Outpatient Pilot Program (LOPPP) were negotiated with representatives of the hospitals (Ontario Ministry of Health n.d.).

The goals of the LOPPP were to optimize the use of spare capacity in hospitals, decrease the flow of outpatient work away from hospitals and collect data on the cost of using hospitals to provide community services. The program, in which twenty hospitals participated, compared laboratory use in a pre-pilot period to a pilot period, during which the hospitals could bring in extra community work and be paid at 75 percent of the OHIP rate for all work done. Regional statistics on overall laboratory use and physician referrals were kept. The pilot was to run for a year, but difficulties starting it and an unexplained abrupt ending meant that most hospitals were only involved for eight or nine months.

The Ministry's evaluation of the LOPPP identified significant methodological problems: it lacked an adequate method for tracking whether work shifted from the private sector to the public sector, and it was difficult to measure the change in cost to the Ministry. Finally, the Ministry noted: "In order to facilitate major workload changes it may have been preferable to have had a longer time frame" (Ontario Ministry of Health n.d.: 14).

Independent evaluation of the program is difficult. The Ministry's final evaluation was only released after a Freedom of Information request, and most of the numbers relating to the private sector were deleted despite the fact they were likely aggregated figures that did not identify individual companies or physicians. The final report shows that all but three of the twenty hospitals had increases in community laboratory work volume and equivalent or greater increases in physician referrals than private labs did. This pattern is a change from the previous ten years, when the growth in private laboratory use far exceeded the increases in hospital volumes. Numerous examples were cited in which hospital marginal cost increases "were below the rate paid by OHIP to private labs" (Ontario Ministry of Health n.d.: 11). None were reported as higher. The LOPPP may not have produced the best data, but it is clear that hospitals, given a financial incentive, could increase their volume of community work, that physicians would use the service and that it would cost less.

The LOPPP worked especially well in Sudbury because the hospital went out and actively recruited community laboratory work. It set up community collection stations that were convenient to doctors' offices and it invested in a transportation system. "We [the hospital] made lots of money … [and] we made a dent in the work going to the private labs," recollects Dr. Bonin, a pathologist at Laurentian Hospital during that time (2006, personal communication). And because the LOPPP rules stipulated that when payments to hospitals exceeded costs, the difference was to be split fifty-fifty with the province, the Ministry saved about $103,000 during the nine months of the Laurentian Hospital experiment. These figures are even more impressive when it is noted that these benefits came from the referrals of only nine community physicians (Forbes 1996).

The limited, if positive, results are partially due to the fact that for both doctors and hospitals, the lack of long-term commitment to the program probably decreased the likelihood of changing referral patterns. This was especially true for hospitals. No money was available to set up community collection networks, and the one hospital that did, Laurentian in Sudbury, was left buying out a lease for a community specimen collection centre it had established when the program suddenly ended. In other words, the hospital was punished for its initiative. Dr. Bonin could not remember why the program was cancelled, but with a strong indication that work was shifting from the for-profit laboratories to hospitals and the growing influence of the corporate sector on government policy, the threat to private profit was likely the reason.

Despite the data in the provincial evaluation report, its conclusion found "mixed results" of cost savings and volume increases. This finding is inexplicable except in the context of the increased power of the for-profit laboratories and the decreased government support for non-profit solutions. The Ministry's faulty evaluation of the LOPPP was used four years later to defend its increased reliance on for-profit laboratories: "Although it appeared that some hospitals were able to increase their performance of out-patient laboratory tests at an apparent lower cost per unit than is currently paid by OHIP, the evaluation of the project yielded mixed results and no firm conclusions were drawn."[27]

Summary

The Ontario provincial government's cost control pressures and problems with for-profit laboratories spurred the growth of non-profit solutions such as the HICL and HHSLP.

The end of the anti-inflation program in 1978 marked the beginning of a significant shift in the provincial government's approach to providing health care services. A memo from Dennis Timbrell, then minister of health, to hospitals and other ministry funded agencies stated:

> Much of the problem for past inflationary pressures has been attributed to increases in the costs of public programs.... The role of the public sector in the economic process has changed fundamentally. We are entering a period of reduced government growth accompanied by a greater recognition of the need to stimulate the growth of the private sector.[28]

This contextual shift, grounded in a global realignment of economic power designed to undercut collective solutions, made it harder to shut down the commercial laboratories and easier to attack public services.

Nonetheless, by 1990, Ontario had two thriving publicly funded non-profit providers of laboratory services to community patients that used hospital laboratories to process the work at a fraction of the cost of the large for-profit corporations. Yet the next two decades were not kind to these programs or to service integration. As the commercial providers came to dominate government laboratory policies these non-profit programs were brought to an end, which is the story of the next chapter.

Notes

1.   "Ontario Hospital Services Commission Expenditure, For the Ten years 1959 to 1968 Inclusive," Statistical Research Division, Ministry of Health, September 5 1969. AO, RG 10-1-2-135, box 3.

2.   "Laboratory Coordination Program Ottawa–Carleton: Policy Manual," December 15, 1980. AO, RG 10-247, container 1, Acc 28303, B212530.

3.   J.L. Penistan, Director Department of Pathology, Stratford General Hospital, "Inter-

Hospital Laboratory Service," October 1971. AO, RG 10-221-2, file: 267, 331.2.3.

4. "Report of Meeting of the Task Force on Laboratory Services," Ontario Council of Health, January 19, 1981. AO, RG 10-247, container 1, Acc 28303, B212530.

5. "Report of a Meeting of the Sub-Committee on Laboratory Systems," Ontario Council of Health, July 27, 1970, item 98. AO RG 10-6-0-27, box 4.

6. "Integration of Hospital Laboratory Services in St. Catherines," August 22, 1967. AO, RG 10-221-2, file: 531.

7. When this project was started it was called In-Common Laboratory and changed its name to HICL in 1974. It will be referred to throughout as HICL.

8. In the last round of regionalization the HHSLP changed its name to the Hamilton Regional Laboratory Medicine Program.

9. "In-Common Laboratory – Toronto," October 13, 1971. AO, RG 10-231-2, file: 266, 531.2.1a.

10. "Regionalization of Hospital Laboratory Services: A Brief Prepared by the Executive of the Section on Clinical Pathology of the Ontario Medical Association," Board Reference #767-1(12.69), January 20, 1970. AO, RG 10-221-2, file: 531.

11. Executive Committee Minutes, OHSC, Feb 5-6, 1969, item 2958. AO, RG 10-45, box 4, B25889, 1969.

12. PPAC Minutes, April 22, 1974, item 5. AO, RG10-45, box 4, B258889, D1974.

13. PPAC Minutes, May 9, 1974, item 3. AO, RG10-45, box 4, B258889, D1974.

14. Winifred Millar letter to William Davis, MPP, September 30, 1976. AO, RG 10-39, file: Laboratory Inspection – Letters of Application, 1976.

15. R.M. McLuckie, Chairman of the Board, HICL, letter to G. Chatfield, Assistant Deputy Minister of Health, June 22, 1976. AO.

16. "Ministers Briefing Book: Laboratory Services Branch," May 21, 1985, p. 49. AO, RG-39, box 5, B383120.

17. "Bulk Billings for Hospital Out-Patient Radiology," February 5, 1974. AO, RG 10-18, barcode 112932, box 2, file 7-47/75(H).

18. "Re: Hospitals In-Common Laboratory Inc.," Memo from C.L. Brubacher, Provincial Laboratory Services Coordinator, to Dr. D. Surplis, Special Assistant to the Minister of Health, April 10, 1981. AO.

19. Minutes of the Sub-Committee on Laboratory Systems, Ontario Council of Health, Nov. 6, 1969. AO, RG 10-6-0-27, box 4.

20. "Capital Equipment costs – Hamilton Regional Laboratories," OHSC/OHIC Executive committee minutes, June 21, 1972, item 4513. AO, RG 10-221-2, file: 268, 531.2.4.

21. "Report on the meeting of the Task Force on Laboratory Services," Ontario Council of Health, November 30, 1981. AO, RG 10-247, container 1, Acc 28303, B212530.

22. "Laboratory Services–Kapuskasing," August 1, 1973. AO, RG 10-18, barcode 112932, box 2, file: 75/73.

23. Letter from J.D. Greig, Chairman, Laboratory Service Committee, Brant District Health Council, to Milton Orris, Area Planning Coordinator, Ministry of Health, March 8, 1977. AO.

24. "Laboratory Co-ordination Activities as of June, 1978," report attached to a memo from M. Fournier to Dr. Aldis, June 26, 1978. The comments on the Niagara, Mississauga, Hanover, Trenton, Peterborough, and Lennox and Addington County Hospitals were all taken from this report. AO.

25. Management Committee Minutes, MOH, June 12, 1976. AO, RG 10-18, Box 15, B156793.

26. Management Committee Minutes, MOH, February 24, 1976. AO, RG 10-18, Box 15, B156793.

27. "Globe and Mail Request for Interview on Private Laboratories," Laboratory Services Branch, May 8, 1984. AO, RG 10-39, box 5, b383120.

28. Dennis Timbrell, Ontario Minister of Health, Memo to: Hospitals and Other Ministry Funded Agencies, June 8, 1978. AO.

Chapter 4

For-Profits Consolidate Power, 1990–2010

The year 1990 marked a turning point in the consolidation of corporate power over community medical laboratories in Ontario. The global capital market, an integrated global economy and its corresponding political movement, neo-liberalism, were sweeping the world. Canada signed the North American Free Trade Agreement, the General Agreement on Trade in Services was completed and the World Trade Organization was formed. Free trade pressures on national and provincial governments encouraged privatization, deregulation and private capital accumulation.

In the twenty-two years since the introduction of medicare, for-profit laboratories had grown both in size and in market share to the point where they effectively controlled Ontario's community laboratory services and were making their first forays into delivering inpatient services. The 1990s saw these laboratories gain real political power. There was a profound shift from the Conservative governments of the1960s and 1970s, which supported the use of hospitals and other non-profit agencies to deliver laboratory services, to the governments since 1990, which have embraced the domination of the for-profits, even using them as an advertisement for increasing private delivery of other health care services.

This chapter examines how, after 1990, Ontario's for-profit laboratories consolidated their political and economic power. The surprise election of an NDP government under Premier Bob Rae in Ontario in 1990 coincided with a recession (lasting from 1989 to 1992) and a rapid increase in the provincial deficit. The Rae government chose the reduction of services as their solution to the fiscal crisis. The $1 billion spent annually on medical laboratory services came under intense scrutiny. Payments to the for-profit laboratories had risen 12 percent per year in the 1980s (Ontario Ministry of Health 1993a), with utiliza-tion increasing faster in the community sector than in hospitals, especially after 1989, when the number of hospital tests peaked.

This chapter starts with an examination of how the reductions in funding for laboratory services effectively reduced costs. The large for-profit corporations were compensated for their lost income with an increase in political power. The election of the Mike Harris Progressive Conservatives in 1995, and subsequent Liberal governments, further rewarded the large companies with a reduction in economic risk and increase in income.

In an effort to find long-term solutions for the laboratory sector, the Rae government established the Laboratory Services Review (LSR). The LSR set in a motion a series of restructuring and integration initiatives that, over the next fifteen years, ended non-profit delivery of community laboratory services and created opportunities, even if they met with limited success, for the private labs to profit from inpatient work.

The Agreement with the OAML

Under budget pressures and faced with out-of-control community laboratory costs, Bob Rae's NDP government took the unprecedented step of negotiating directly with the Ontario Association of Medical Laboratories (OAML) to establish policies and payments for community laboratory services. Previously, OHIP payments for community laboratory services had been negotiated between the MOH, the OMA and the OAML.

This was not the pattern followed in British Columbia and Manitoba, where the doctors' professional associations still negotiate on behalf of the private laboratories. The sidelining of the OMA in Ontario probably relates to the size and commercialization of the industry and the increasing influence of the OAML, which primarily represented the interests of the largest laboratory corporations. Even before this negotiation, the OAML had begun to deal "directly with senior MOH officials on contentious issues" (Ontario Ministry of Health 1993a). At the same time, many pathologists in public hospitals supported a greater role for hospitals in providing community laboratory work, directly countering one of the main political goals of the OAML. This resulted in hostility from the OAML, witnessed in 1997 when it refused to let the OMA laboratory section send a representative to an OAML committee because it could "serve only a political agenda and that not the OAML's."[1]

This new bi-party relationship was acknowledged in the 1993 Memorandum of Understanding between the OAML and the MOH (Ontario Ministry of Health 1993d), which limited the fee-for-service system by imposing, for the first time, a hard cap on funding for the sector. The for-profit labs still billed on a per-test basis, but their overall income was capped at a share, equal to their market share, of the total funding allocated to the sector. Rather than focusing on increasing utilization, the commercial sector now had to balance attracting business with limiting access to make sure that the amount of service provided did not exceed what they would be paid for.

The Memorandum also set up committees to administer private laboratory licensing, develop laboratory policy, negotiate the fee schedule and examine utilization. The OAML had input on all policies affecting laboratories, including those in hospitals, while the OHA and the OMA had limited input into policies that dealt directly with the for-profit laboratories. This created an influence imbalance that favoured the private sector. The OMA continued to be in charge of quality control through the Laboratory Proficiency Testing Program (LPTP).

The Memorandum also established a secure funding base for the industry's lobbying arm, the OAML. A Rand-like formula was set up; the government withheld $500,000 per year from payments to the private labs and transferred it to the OAML, a system which was ongoing in 2010. The government also agreed to pay $10.5 million over three years (1993–1996) into a slush fund for the commercial laboratories for research and to help with restructuring.

Equally profitably labs in Alberta asked for $13 million, and in British Columbia pathologists wanted $60 million when their fees were cut to control costs. In all cases the funds were to be provided by the public and controlled by the private sector. A key goal in Ontario was funding research to enhance the industry's export potential. The Memorandum implies that most of the research results would be proprietary information, further discouraging integration among the commercial laboratories. The fund has been described by an industry insider as a "sop to MDS" (Sutherland 2007: 136), a government favourite. I asked the Ministry for details of how these funds were spent, but no records were provided. By 1995, $8 million had been dispersed from the fund.

Since the first memorandum signed between the NDP government and the OAML, the Ministry has continued to negotiate funding for community laboratory services in private with the for-profit corporations. The resulting agreements cover not only detailed fee setting and total funding for the sector, but also incentives for complying with regionalization initiatives, changes to the discount system, the locating of specimen collection centres, what tests and technologies are to be publicly covered, policies on the non-profit providers, services to underserviced areas and nursing homes and interpretations of regulations. In 2000, the OAML felt it had good access to the MOH, boasting of a 40 percent increase in consultations with Ministry staff on a wide range of issues.[2]

The intent of the Memorandum was to "support the continuing viability of a restructured commercial laboratory industry" (Ontario Ministry of Health 1993d), which it did. And, while the Memorandum did recognize the possibility that the LSR might transfer work to or from hospitals, the strengthened private system made it harder both politically and financially to transfer work to the public sector.

Large Labs Respond to Hard Caps with Service Cuts

The Memorandum's short-term effect on cost control was as profound as its political effects: payments for community laboratory work actually dropped in the four years after 1993. Simply capping funding for community laboratory services left it to the for-profit corporations to decide where the cuts would be made, which often meant a reduction in access for smaller communities and marginalized patients. In 1994, both MDS and CML sent letters to family doctors and patients advising them that free in-home specimen collection would no longer be available; a user fee would now be charged for this service. Collection services in doctors' offices were restricted, forcing patients to go to collection centres or hospitals to have their blood taken (Nicol and Nolan 1998). Physicians reported concern that many of the incentives that had facilitated access and reduced their costs, such as laboratories renting space in medical buildings, supplying phlebotomists to doctors' offices and providing supplies, were being cancelled (Thorburn 1999). Similarly, there was a reduction in service to nursing home residents until the government negotiated an agreement in 1999 that included extra money for the private laboratories to provide service to these patients. In 1999, when Med-Chem, Ontario's fourth largest laboratory, went bankrupt, physicians reported difficulty finding other laboratories to service their patients because, "there appears to be a significant lack of inducement to accept new business" (Thorburn 1999: 24).

The commercial laboratories also participated in programs aimed at decreasing utilization by changing the way physicians ordered tests. In the early 1990s, the OAML produced guidelines for physicians that were effective in reducing laboratory utilization (van Walraven, Vivek and Chan 1998; Bunting and van Walraven 2003). In the era of hard caps, companies were more receptive than they had been in the 1970s to programs limiting utilization, though it needs to be noted that after 1998 when revenue caps increased the volume of laboratory work started to climb again. Starting in 2005, the agreements with the OAML included new money beyond the caps to compensate for increased volume.

The funding caps marked a shift in laboratory expenditure patterns. In 1991, for-profit laboratories accounted for 48 percent of all laboratory expenditures; by 2005 this had dropped to 41 percent. The caps worked. Following two decades in which expenditures for community laboratory work rose twice as quickly as hospital spending, hospitals started to consume more of the province's medical laboratory budget. From 1997 to 2005, for the first time, the number of tests in hospitals and hospital laboratory expenditures rose faster than in the for-profit laboratories

With the introduction of the hard caps, the for-profit laboratories cut many of the less profitable services, reduced access, closed many laboratories and focused more on the high-volume, less-expensive tests. Hospitals on the other hand have had an increase in test diversity, with many more complex and expensive tests (Ontario Hospital Association 2000), such as cancer pathology testing, on a greater percentage of sicker patients who they are required to see. Despite reductions in some small hospitals, the public sector, as part of its mandate to provide services to all parts of the province, continues to maintain extensive province-wide facilities, including laboratory services to many smaller communities, which carries a higher cost. Also, the increase in hospital laboratory volume probably reflects the larger number of patients being seen in a shorter

Table 4-1   Expenditure on Laboratory Services by Ownership, 1972–2006
              (actual dollars)

	72–75	75–81	81–91	91–97	97–06
For-profit	218%	67%	283%	4%	30%
Hospital	53%	54%	147%	8%	80%

Source: 1972–1981, Minster's Briefing Book: Laboratory Services Branch," May 21, 1985, p. 22. AO, RG-39, box 5, B383120; 1991, (Ontario Ministry of Health 1993e); 1997–2005, Laboratories Branch of the Ministry of Health.

time as hospital work shifts to expedited discharges, outpatient clinics and day surgeries (Ontario Hospital Association 2000). This shift in utilization patterns will require more study but it goes a long way to explaining why expenditures on Ontario hospitals have increased despite the entrenchment of neoliberal health care policies.

While the big labs responded to funding caps by cutting services, the smaller for-profits became more responsive to community needs. They filled gaps left by the major conglomerates, increasing their market share and thus their share of the funding. Simultaneously, hospitals, particularly smaller hospitals, were looking for ways to maintain their laboratory services and make some money to offset reductions in government funding.

From 1990 to 1996, the HICL opened thirteen new specimen collection centres, most in partnership with smaller community hospitals. This compares to eight, including the head office, opened between 1978 and 1989. The LSR's evaluation of the HICL indicates some of the reasons for this success:

> HICL has demonstrated that, by providing a common logistic network for specimen collection, specimen transportation and test reporting, sharing arrangements between laboratories can be beneficial, leading to improved volume of testing, automation and increased efficiency. (Ontario Ministry of Health 1994a: 12)

The 1992 Laboratory Services Review

The Memorandum with the OAML found a short-term solution to the increasing costs of laboratory services, but because the Rae government was also interested in finding a long-term solution to the sector's difficulties, the NDP established the Laboratory Services Review in 1992 to find these systemic answers. The LSR was the third large public evaluation of the laboratory sector in as many decades. The review took place in a political climate of heightened concern about government expenditures and a rapidly changing health care system. The shift to more outpatient clinics, day surgeries and home care for the acutely ill created a greater demand for the sharing of test results. New computer technologies raised the possibility of increased integration, and advances in point-of-care testing, i.e., testing specimens at the bedside or in the community, led to questions about the need for more centralized laboratory work.

Diana Schatz, a microbiologist and founder of the Michener Institute, was chosen to head the LSR. She worked with an external advisory committee composed of representatives from unions, for-profit corporations, hospitals, professional organizations and the HICL. The LSR continued a long tradition of studying the laboratory sector and being bedevilled by its divisions. The report starts off with a caveat that recommendations on utilization, cost and system development were limited by difficulties in comparing the hospital and community sectors. These technical incompatibilities were mirrored in the political debate between those who supported the for-profits and those who favoured more public, non-profit solutions. In fact, the for-profit versus non-profit debate and the related funding issues became the defining issues in the province-wide public hearings on the LSR's draft report.

While these tensions between sectors had been evident in the 1982 Ontario Council on Health Task Force on Laboratory Services, they were of secondary interest. The for-profit providers were not represented on the task force, and its conclusions assumed that the non-profit system would dominate and commercial labs would be peripheral players.

The pro-market forces portrayed the LSR and its outcomes as a test of how anti-business the NDP government would be. At the Toronto hearings Martin Barkin, a former deputy minister of health and director of Gamma-Dynacare Medical Laboratories (GDML), issued an implied threat: "Private investors are watching laboratory reform as an indicator of the general investment climate for health industries in Ontario."[3] This theme was reinforced by MDS CEO John Rogers, who argued for the many benefits of profits, including increased tax revenues, creation of wealth and jobs, development of new technologies for export and increased investment in the province by health care companies.[4]

Background reports commissioned by the LSR show a bias towards commercialization of the sector, likely reflecting the bias of the Ministry's bureaucracy, which was responsible for contracting the studies. Two of five studies, the ones on information technology and system delivery (GSA Consulting 1993; CLS and GSA Consulting 1994), were written by a U.S. firm involved in managing hospital laboratories, many of them for-profit, and marketing laboratory services. They suggest that the hospital laboratory of the future will be commercialized and integrated with the private sector. The other background documents were basic descriptions of the existing system and written in Ontario.

Supporters of greater use of the public sector talked about how the current funding arrangements harmed hospitals, kept costs high and defeated system goals such as maintaining or improving quality and the efficient use of human resources. Most advocated for a level playing field between the hospitals and the commercial laboratories on which they could compete for the community work. A few argued for the more radical position that all the work be transferred to the public sector.

LSR: No Decisions a Private Victory

Commenting on her report, Dr. Schatz (2006, personal communication) said that the LSR avoided taking positions on funding because of irreconcilable differences within the advisory committee. Instead the recommendations supported devolution of planning to districts, which would then work out solutions involving all of the partners, both for-profit and non-profit. Regional plans would build on the twenty-five hospital-based cooperative efforts that already existed. No community laboratory initiatives were mentioned. Although more accepting of the existence of the for-profit sector, these recommendations were very similar to those that came out of the 1970 and the 1982 Ontario Council on Health task forces. The problems remained but the shift in power to capital in the global economy allowed more for-profit involvement.

The headline in the *Toronto Star* on the release of the LSR summed up reactions and foretold the direction of laboratory services over the next decade: "Provincial report backs private labs: Industry relieved, health care unions furious" (Chamberlain 1994, D1). It is not so much that the report backed private labs as that it accepted their continued existence, and it made no recommendations to increase the use of hospital labs. This was a victory for the private laboratories because they were now firmly recognized as a central part of the system. The unions objected to the conclusions and, along with the HICL, refused to endorse the report.

The LSR decision to leave the for-profit companies alone dovetailed nicely with the NDP's industrial strategy of developing strong Ontario industries that could compete in the international marketplace. The Health Industry Advisory Council set up by the NDP advocated using domestic markets as a "springboard to developing globally competitive health industry companies."[5] MDS's Canadian roots and links to the NDP made it an ideal candidate for a local company that could receive government support to be a winner internationally. In practical terms this meant more access to hospital laboratories for private management services, help restructuring and more for-profit-hospital joint ventures with new technologies such as MDS's AutoLab (Ontario Ministry of Health 1993c).

The election of an NDP government in 1990 had been a cause for hope among hospital laboratory workers. Under increasingly tight hospital budgets, laboratory staff became concerned about job security, and hospitals, particularly smaller hospitals, were concerned about maintaining the volume needed for adequate laboratory services. On the other hand the for-profit laboratories were wary of the socialists: they were convinced that the government was intent on shutting them down. As much as some would have liked to see this, there is nothing in the written record to indicate that this was ever the government's intention.

The NDP was more intent on establishing its credentials as a government for "all of Ontario," by finding short-term solutions to the province's budget problems and developing long-term solutions that would show them to be good managers. The result was a willful blindness to the real problems in laboratory services, which amounted to encouragement for the for-profit sector. This blindness was reinforced by the size of the commercial labs. They implied that there would be significant political fallout from job loss, declining stock values and reduced economic growth if they were harmed. Also, harming the for-profit laboratories would undercut the NDP's economic strategy of finding "winners" in the health care field. The private laboratories emerged from the rule of Ontario's first social democratic government in a stronger position.

Regulation 02/98 — Ending Competition

When the industry funding cap, HICL expansion and the increasingly aggressive smaller laboratories started to threatened the profits of larger laboratories, they responded by using the OAML to negotiate with the government to limit competition for community laboratory services. The newly elected Mike Harris Conservative government was glad to oblige. Harris had close ties to GDML, one the largest for-profit companies, and was prepared to go against his stated free-market principles and work with the OAML to secure the financial position of the large lab companies.

In 1998, the Conservatives introduced Regulation 02/98, an amendment to Regulation 552 of the *Health Insurance Act*, which fixed the division of the funding cap between existing companies on the basis of their market share in 1996. This regulation closely resembled a proposal drafted by OAML lawyers and sent to the Ministry for approval in March 1997.[6] These changes made it virtually impossible for a new company to start up or for a company's market share to increase unless it merged with another firm.

GDML argued that the regulation was developed as a solution to problems caused by the NDP's cuts and that it would use taxpayers' money wisely for "patient services and testing," rather than fighting for market share (*Toronto Star* 1999). It was supported as a cost control measure that would improve service. But cost control was clearly not the concern of the larger labs. Costs had fallen through the first half of the 1990s and only started to increase again after the 1998 regulation came into effect. Protection of their market share and income was what the big companies wanted. A review of Regulation 02/98 by the federal Competition Bureau found that it "would reduce the incentive to provide good service and would have the effect of suppressing competition on service levels, quality, turnaround time and reliability" (Donovan 1998). Regulation 02/98 was written by the larger for-profit labs for their own benefit.

After 1998, competition between laboratories shifted from fighting for market share by increasing service to fighting for more money from the government, cutting costs to increase profits and merging. In 1999, Med-Chem Health Care, the fourth largest laboratory in Ontario, went bankrupt after going "deeply in debt to finance an ambitious acquisition plan" (Greenwood 1999). Analysts were quoted as saying that the potential buyers were more interested in the company's business contracts, a large one being its share of Ontario's laboratory market, than in its facilities or employees. Med-Chem was purchased by CML, which further concentrated the sector (Cole 2004).

Regulation 02/98 was the end point of a convoluted policy-market dynamic in the laboratory sector in the 1990s. Government cost controls had increased competition, which helped the smaller laboratories and hurt the larger ones. The big labs then worked with government to end competition, penalize the small labs and make Ontario's community medical laboratory market one of the more tightly controlled in the Canadian economy.

The Failed Long-Term Solution — Regional Integration

Concurrent with cutting funding, the NDP government started what they hoped would bring long-term solutions to the problems in laboratory services.

Immediately following the release of the LSR in 1994, the NDP minister of health established the Ontario Laboratory Services Implementation Secretariat (OL-SIS), the first in a series of regionalization efforts, all of which were doomed to failure. The importance of understanding this policy history is that it shows the privileged position of private companies in government policy implementation: a consistent pattern of for-profit companies sabotaging government policy for their own benefit is revealed, and, simultaneously, the public sector proves itself to be better at working with government policy.

Round 1 — Regional Laboratory Committees

In 1996, the OLSIS brought together providers, professionals and policy-makers in nine regions to develop integration plans. The goal was to take advantage of the strengths of the public and private sectors through "effective partnerships." The services to be integrated included specimen transfer, management, purchasing, human resources and patient information (Ontario Ministry of Health 1996), all services that could easily be contracted to for-profit providers, and that started to happen. There was no mention of making maximum use of laboratory facilities. There was a feeling in the laboratory community that regional plans would be in place by the end of 1996.[7] The OLSIS had, at best, uneven results and in the end it was put on hold and an attempt was made to force laboratory integration through a request for proposals (RFP) process.

Round 2 — Regional RFPs: Failed Forced Integration

The lacklustre performance of the OLSIS was followed by a more forceful approach to integration. After a series of consultations in the summer of 1998,[8] from which the unions were excluded,[9] and an internal study by consultants Coopers and Lybrand (1997), the Ministry decided to ask for RFPs in three regions to deliver all the laboratory services, inpatient and community, for a fixed envelope of funding based on current laboratory expenses. This approach removed the government from directly setting the funding of hospitals or for-profit labs, or from forcing hospitals to make greater use of the for-profit sector. The government simply set rules for the RFP and told the providers to work it out. This approach strongly resembled a recommendation put forward two years before by Paul Gould (1997), CEO of the OAML, when he argued that companies should competitively bid for a contract to provide all the laboratory services in a designated area. In support of his argument he referred to a publication by the Fraser Institute, a right-wing think tank committed to the privatization of health services. A similar approach had been taken by the Klein government in Alberta in 1995.

The first RFP was issued in January 1999. Bidders had to be licensed providers already in the system, and both public and private sector providers had to be involved in the consortium submitting the proposal. The contracts were to be for five years. It is important to understand how this process limited possible alternatives. It precluded what many would argue would be the lowest cost and most integrated of possible solutions: a consortium of hospitals developing a non-profit body like the HICL to organize collection of community laboratory specimens for processing in hospital laboratory facilities.

The RFP was withdrawn because none of the proposals met the minimum requirements. For-profit companies were concerned about what would happen to their fixed costs, such as rent, if they should lose the bid and how the outcome of the RFP process would affect their contracts with the government guaranteeing them payment for a certain market share. Hospitals complained that there was not enough time to develop a full proposal.[10] A 2004 recommendation in British Columbia to use a similar competitive bidding process was withdrawn after an outcry from both the private and the public providers. Alberta's 1995 attempt also failed initially, only succeeding when Premier Ralph Klein forced the major private labs in Edmonton and Calgary into partnerships (Ballerman 2010, personal communication).

In the evaluation meeting that followed the collapse of the RFP process in Ontario, both the OHA and the OAML rejected the competitive process. Instead they favoured a facilitated process driven by the current providers and building on their interests. The OAML was the most anxious to return to a voluntary regional laboratory strategy. It emphasized that hospitals and commercial laboratories should be recognized as the primary providers in the sectors they currently control (Page and Kornovski 2000). While the benefits of competition might have been fundamental to the belief system of those arguing for more for-profit services, the RFP process highlighted the threats to for-profit providers posed by a competitive, integrated system.

Round 3 — Facilitated Hospital Integration for Private Profit

The program that emerged from the ashes of the RFP was the Ontario Regional Laboratory Services Planning (ORLSP), implemented in October 2000. It was organized in the same nine regions as previous restructuring efforts. The process was facilitated by consultants from THiiNC Health Care — the same company that had been contracted by the BC government in its laboratory restructuring process and one with a strong history of supporting public-private partnerships. THiiNC brought together representatives of the OMA (laboratory physicians), the OAML (commercial laboratories) and the OHA (hospital laboratories) to develop regional plans for hospital and community laboratory services that would ensure accessibility, limit duplication of operations and services, meet quality standards and ensure "an appropriate critical mass where testing is performed."[11]

Hospital representation on the regional steering committees (RSC) of the ORLSP process was regional, but the private laboratories opted for a province-wide approach. CML and GDML had the same person representing their interests on six RSCs. MDS had two people covering three each and an extra representative on the Toronto RSC. The private labs had broader corporate interests than simply improving services in a region. They were interested in moving work to their centralized facilities. Also, the commercial providers had a province-wide agreement that left them with very little interest in developing regional arrangements that might affect their provincial market share.

The ORLSP did facilitate some new hospital integration, for instance, microbiology services in the Central West region, and it furthered others that had started in the 1960s and 70s, for instance, in Hamilton, Kingston, Ottawa, Stratford and the Northwest. The Eastern Ontario Regional Laboratory Association (EORLA) is by far the most aggressive of these integration initiatives. It aims to bring ownership of laboratory services in all the hospitals around Ottawa under one non-profit company. The corporation is controlled by representatives from area hospitals and the board includes members of the public served and laboratory specialists. GDML was contracted to help design, build and manage Ottawa's regional hospital laboratory.

Once again the central role of a for-profit company raises questions of conflict of interest. "The model for delivery of laboratory services in EORLA will be closer to the private laboratory service delivery model, and like the private sector, operational and financial best practices will be key to success" (QSE Consulting 2006: 4). While it is not clear what this means on a day-to-day basis, it does mean less redundancy in the system, fewer highly trained staff and less service at smaller rural hospitals. If the system is undersized, a complaint levelled against the regional laboratory in Ottawa (Jenson 2007, personal communication) and if adequate allowances have not been made for surges in work, surges inherent in any hospital system, or for base increases in volume, then it may be necessary for the overflow to be sent to a private laboratory: possibly the GDML lab in Ottawa. Removing excess capacity from the hospital system limits the possibility of further integration of community laboratory work with hospitals.

Regionalization can either harm or benefit patient services depending on how it is planned and implemented. Are the recommendations from GDML the best for regional inpatient laboratory services? Or are they best for protecting GDML's community market? Did GDML design and manage the regional laboratory to ensure regular use of the GDML lab?

The main differences between the regionalization initiatives hospitals took in the 1960s and those in 1995–2010 are that now the process was being forced by the government and the private sector had to be involved. It is unclear, though, whether the presence of the for-profit laboratories did little other than help them identify ways they could sell their services to hospitals or more effectively compete with hospitals. For example, when the private laboratories came to regional steering committee meetings, they were not required to produce reports, as was mandatory for the hospitals (Sutherland 2007). This unequal participation allowed the private labs to gain good knowledge of hospital plans, helping them identify opportunities to bid on hospital work and introduce programs that would undercut hospital initiatives.

Regionalization Results

After fifteen years of regionalization initiatives, little if any progress has been made on limiting duplication between community and inpatient laboratory services in Ontario. Most communities have one hospital network and two or three competing community providers, often with specimen collection stations across the street from each other.

For forty years, governments have sought to integrate Ontario's laboratory system. Despite tens of millions of dollars of financial incentives promised to the private sector if they gave their full support to the various integration initiatives, success has been limited. Hospitals received no specific extra funding and contributed much more to the effort. In 2006, the OHA identified fifteen regional hospital-based laboratory information systems (Ontario Hospital e-Health Council 2006). The disparate interests of the hospitals and the for-profit providers, public service versus private profit, plus the government for-profit bias, helped keep the two systems separate.

The Real Government Policy

At the same time as the laboratory section of the Ontario Ministry of Health was spending a lot of money and time trying to integrate services, other government initiatives worked to separate hospital and community systems.

The Hospital Services Restructuring Commission (HSRC), created in 1996, quickly came into conflict with the laboratory initiatives. The HSRC created a situation in which the hospitals often did not know what their future governance structure was going to be. This made it difficult for them to negotiate regional laboratory integration. The HSRC was also integrating services in regions with different boundaries than the nine laboratory restructuring regions. The government made no effort to coordinate these parallel processes involving overlapping but different sets of laboratories within overlapping but different sets of boundaries.

A similar structural barrier to planning and integration was created in 2004 when Dalton McGuinty's Liberal government established the Local Health Integration Networks (LHINs), a regional structure for delivering health services. The LHINs, which are organized on fourteen regions instead of the nine used by the Laboratories Branch, are charged with rationalizing some health services in a region, including hospital laboratory services, but the community laboratory sector is excluded from their mandate. A hospital laboratory specialist commented that the LHINs added "another level of chaos" to the medical laboratory system (Sutherland 2007: 133). Along with maintaining a structural division between hospitals and community laboratories, including different funding and administrative regimes, the LHINs reinforce an old tension that works against public-sector delivery. The LHINs have a fixed budget to deliver the health care services within their mandate. If the cost of hospital laboratory services can be reduced, the money can be shifted to other services. At the same time, since the community laboratory sector is paid from a different budget, one that is negotiated directly between the for-profit laboratories and the government, and permits some payment increases as workload increases, the for-profit labs can benefit from absorbing off-loaded hospital services. The additional spending on for-profit services will not affect the LHINs' budgets, but it will increase the Ministry's budget.

Divisions between the inpatient and community services were strengthened in 2000 when the OMA took over negotiating with the MOH on behalf of the hospital pathologists and reached a province-wide agreement increasing pay and improving working conditions.[12] On the other hand, the OMA Laboratory Medicine Section described the situation of fee-for-service doctors employed in the commercial sector as "deplorable"[13] and complained regularly about the discounting system used by the for-profit laboratories to reduce payment to the pathologists.

It is hard to avoid the conclusion, because the outcomes are so stark, that despite its rhetoric and the millions of dollars spent on the regionalization of laboratory services, Ontario's real government policy was to maintain separate systems except where it was profitable for commercial laboratories to provide inpatient services. After forty years of policy to integrate services and fifteen years of concentrated regionalization programs, community laboratory services are more clearly separated from inpatient laboratory services than ever.

Reduction in Non-Profit Community Lab Services

In the first decade of the twenty-first century, the drive of the for-profits for complete domination of the community sector has continued unabated. Hospitals, under pressure from the LHINs to cut costs, have made a strategic financial decision to stop providing community laboratory services. Invariably this has meant a shift of work to for-profit laboratories. Events in Cornwall indicate how hard these changes may be to track. The hospital there closed its community laboratory services and shifted the work to a non-profit community health clinic. The clinic then contracted GDML to collect and process the work (More 2006/2007).

Closing hospitals to community patients has increased inequities in the system. Traditionally, hospitals have provided an equity safety valve in that they have usually processed uninsured tests ordered by doctors at no cost to patients. Now those who cannot pay will have to go without. Until recently one common uninsured test that was done in hospitals for community patients was the PSA. When hospitals stopped providing this service, the province started, under some conditions, to cover the cost, increasing the income of the private labs: a benefit that had been denied to the hospitals.

The HICL has also shrunk. In 1996, the HICL, as the result of an agreement between the MOH and the OAML, was informed by the Ministry that it would have to end all of its community laboratory services by January 1997. Closing the HICL's community work ended $11 million in payments to hospital laboratories and was one more pressure forcing hospitals into partnerships with for-profit laboratories (Watts 1997).

The potential devastation from closing the HICL's community services, especially to small hospitals, led to a spirited province-wide coalition of unions, hospitals, pathologists and public health care activists. Their campaign produced a partial victory. The Ministry was forced to allow twelve small hospitals, in nine "pilot projects," to enter into joint ventures with partners who would collect community laboratory specimens and have the hospital's laboratory process the work. The HICL became the community partner in six of these pilots, MDS in two and GDML in one. The government agreed to pay the pilot projects 86 percent of the standard OHIP rate for the volume of work performed in 1996. This gross payment stayed the same for the next ten years, despite an increase in workload. The fee-for-service laboratories had their payments increase 36 percent during the same time.

The Ministry hired RPO Consultants to review the pilot projects in 2008. The study found that the communities with pilot projects received faster results, better trained staff stayed in smaller hospitals and per-test costs were less. Despite these advantages the pilot projects ran counter to the "provincial model of testing" favoured by the Ministry and the commercial laboratories for community laboratory work, so they were terminated. The exclusion of the for-profit laboratories from the LHINs became a reason for LHINs' management to shut down these pilot projects, transferring community work from small hospital laboratories to the corporate laboratories.

In 2010, the HICL transferred its last community specimen collection centre to a private lab. The HICL still runs "the grid," which coordinates the use of hospital laboratories for esoteric tests, and continues to expand as an internationally recognized referral centre.

The Hamilton Regional Laboratory Medicine Program, another successful community-hospital partnership started in the 1970s, was forced to close its community laboratory services program in the fall of 2007 (Tajaja 2007, personal communication). Once again, the work was shifted to the for-profit corporations.

Contracting Private Services

While the private sector has encroached on inpatient laboratory services, an encroachment only possible because of government policy and funding, its success there has been limited compared to its domination of community services. MDS took its first steps into the hospital sector in the mid-1980s with management contracts for hospitals in the Niagara Peninsula. Many of these arrangements were short-term consulting or "change" contracts. MDS managed laboratory restructuring, which often involved cutting staff and reorganizing along business lines. St. Catherine's General Hospital and the Wellesley Hospital used MDS for similar purposes.

The move into the hospital system started in earnest in the 1990s with the introduction of the hard funding caps. The large for-profit laboratories looking for other sources of income identified the delivery of inpatient services as a significant and potentially lucrative market. As described earlier, GDML played a central role in establishing the Eastern Ontario Regional Laboratory. Numerous requests were made to find out how much GDML was paid for its work and they were not answered. But it is inconceivable that it is less than hundreds of thousands of dollars and it's possibly in the millions.

In 1996, an agreement between the OAML and the MOH allowed the private laboratories to start processing twelve complex esoteric tests that had previously only been done in public hospitals. This change allowed the commercial labs to sell these tests to smaller hospitals and remove some income from larger ones. For instance, in northwestern Ontario, LifeLabs is the main reference laboratory for the smaller hospitals and has a computer interlink with Thunder Bay Regional Hospital's laboratory (Ontario Hospital e-Health Council 2006). This is one of the areas of the province that has a history of the same medical director overseeing both public and private laboratories. Similarly in the Niagara region, LifeLabs has business relationships and shares medical directors with local hospitals.

Joint Ventures

The first joint ventures in Ontario between the lab companies and public hospitals were for non-lab services. MDS started a long relationship with the Toronto Hospital (the old Toronto General and the Wellesley and now a member of the University Health Network) by partnering in 1986 to form Health and Research Services, a company to develop and commercialize orthopedic products and diagnostic testing procedures. GDML set up a joint venture rehabilitation therapy clinic with St. Joseph's Hospital in London (Fuller 1998).

MDS's next big joint venture in Canada was with the Toronto Hospital in 1995 when they formed the Toronto Medical Laboratory (TML) to serve both community patients and inpatients. MDS saw the joint venture as an opportunity to use the hospital site to demonstrate its newly patented automated technology, the AutoLab. This technology had become the poster child for how innovative Canada's commercial laboratories are. The hospital hoped to gain expertise in automation, computer technology and commercialization of research.[14] The hospital continued to own and staff the lab, underwriting most of the operational risk. MDS had limited success selling the AutoLab, but the joint venture helped subsidize its development. MDS did use the technology in its internal operations, and it is part of reason it was able to cut the number of its laboratories in Ontario from twenty-six in 1995 to twelve in 2006.

The TML was dissolved in 2009. All of the laboratory services for the University Hospital Network (UHN), the amalgamated structure including the Toronto General Hospital, Princess Margaret Hospital and the Toronto Western Hospital, have been taken over by the UHN's laboratory medicine program. The TML's last large contract, to provide services to ten hospitals in northeastern Ontario, has been taken over by the UHN. The stand-alone TML lab has been closed, and all the work moved back into the Toronto General Hospital location (Mason 2010, personal communication).

In 1996, Sunnybrook Hospital in Toronto entered into a joint venture with GDML to develop a multipurpose laboratory facility. It has since folded, though there is still some sharing of work between the hospital and the private company.

Brenda Gamble (2002) examined two joint ventures between academic health science hospitals and for-profit laboratory corporations. In these cases the hospitals provided most of the management and hired the staff. Case A, which was not working well at the time of the research, used an automated laboratory technology that was provided by the for-profit corporation. The joint venture was to be a demonstration site for the new technology. The hospital paid 50 percent of the "significant" capital costs. Case B used facilities in the hospital and leased equipment. The hospital in Case B reported a 16 percent saving on laboratory costs, though it is not clear whether this was a result of better management, lower labour costs or community and uninsured work being done in the joint-venture facility. In neither case was Gamble able to verify the costs. In spite of signing a confidentiality agreement, she was not allowed to see any financial statements.

Both of the joint ventures studied by Gamble were intended to become regional laboratories, and neither, at the time of her research, were making progress towards that goal. This led her to comment: "Reform driven by market incentives (i.e., the establishment of commercial laboratories) [her nomenclature describing the new for-profit joint ventures] could result in the fragmentation of services" (Gamble 2002: 120). While the partners in Gamble's joint ventures were not identified, they sound a lot like the joint ventures involving Sunnybrook and the Toronto Hospital.

Other partnerships have also ended. Timmins and District Hospital signed a letter of intent for a partnership with GDML, but this was not pursued after discussions with the laboratory technologists' union.[15] Similarly, MDS entered into a joint venture with the Calgary Regional Health Authority in 1996 to provide all community and hospital laboratory work, but the partnership was bought out by the Health Authority in 2006. The joint venture in Edmonton that saw most routine hospital work shift to offsite private laboratories was reversed in 2006. In the 1990s, MDS approached provincial governments in Manitoba, Saskatchewan, Nova Scotia and New Brunswick with proposals to provide laboratory services, including inpatient and public health services. None of these turned into successful projects.

These failed projects illustrate some of the problems with private companies taking on hospital work. Although looking for larger markets, commercial companies are hesitant about taking on the risks inherent in hospital laboratory work. For instance, "stat" services, fluctuating volume requirements and more individualized testing are anathema to the routinization preferred in industrial laboratories, the mainstay of for-profit laboratory work in Canada. The manager of Kingston General Hospital's laboratory services described the difference between the work of for-profit laboratories and that of hospital laboratories as "routine work compared to custom work," when offering an explanation of the lack of success of commercial provision of inpatient services (More 2010, personal communication).

New Tests and Programs

Like pharmaceuticals, the laboratory industry is actively engaged in creating new products and increasing demand for their services, first in the population, then in the publicly funded health care system. CML, for example, has as one of its key business strategies growing its non-capped revenues, which means selling more tests not covered by Ontario's funding cap. Gamma-Dynacare has been known to pay clinics more money to collect samples that are not publicly financed; the price for these tests is set as high as the market will bear. As the company increases demand, pressure will grow on the government to bring these tests into the publicly funded system.

When new laboratory tests are included in the list of services to be publicly funded, the Ministry must decide a fee-for-service price. The commercial laboratory sector in Ontario has secured from the government a promise to give "due weight" to the concern of the laboratories that the revenue they receive "will not be less favourable than when the test was not insured."[16] Rather than trying to determine a price for a new test based on actual costs the government has made a commitment to take into consideration the private sector price even if it is unreasonably high. While this policy will be reviewed under the terms of the most recent agreement between the OAML and the Ministry, it shows a pandering to private interests over the Ministry's obligation to the public to get the best deal. Ontario's auditor general's 2005 report identified the government's lack of understanding of the real costs of tests when negotiating with the OAML as a problem.

As well as trying to increase demand for new tests, private labs push to increase utilization of more established measures, such as for Vitamin D levels, the fastest growing lab test, and public health surveillance programs that use lab testing, such as fecal occult blood testing. These tests and dozens like them can provide valuable results, but the current levels of use are seriously questioned (Hadler 2004).

The public discussion on what new tests to cover, when they should be used and how much should be paid for them is confounded by the power of a large profitable industry working to shape public and professional opinion as a marketing strategy for their products. As bad as the skewing of the public debate is, salt is rubbed into this wound by the government providing significant tax savings at public expense for many of these corporate activities, such as marketing, lobbying and research and development. The laboratory industry gets to use public money to shape policy for their private benefit with limited, if any, public control.

Summary

The shift in the global economy to more corporate power played itself out in Ontario's laboratory sector with increased political power and economic stability for the large for-profit laboratory corporations. In the twenty years since Rae's NDP government formally recognized the for-profit providers as the key players in the community laboratory sector, barriers between inpatient and community services have hardened to protect the for-profit control of the community laboratory market and softened to permit greater for-profit involvement in the delivery of inpatient services. Government initiatives to promote complete integration have largely been unsuccessful because of industry opposition and overriding government policies that favour for-profit providers.

Commercial laboratories have played an active role in shutting down non-profit services, and government policies have made it easier to transfer work from hospitals to private laboratories. Largely out of the public eye, agreements negotiated between the government and the for-profit industry have provided a lucrative and steady income stream, with consistent dividends to the private shareholders.

In 2007, there were only eleven laboratory corporations in Ontario, and three of these, LifeLabs, CML and GDML, controlled 93 percent of the $592 million community market. The next chapter examines these beneficiaries of Ontario's laboratory polices and what have they done with our money.

Notes

1. Paul Gould, CEO of the OAML, letter to Brian Sheridan, MDS Associate Medical Director, May 16, 1997.
2. Virginia Turner, CEO OAML, "Year 1999–2000 and the Future 2000–2001," speech to the OAML Annual General Meeting, March 29, 2001.
3. Martin Barkin, "Presentation to Lab Services Review," copy of a slide show, n.d.
4. John Rogers, CEO and President of MDS, "Laboratory Services Review Hearings," deputation, January 21, 1994.
5. "Terms of Reference: Health industries Sector Council." Attachment to a letter from Andrew Szende, Head, Health Economic Development, Ministry of Health, to Julie Davis, Secretary Treasurer of the Ontario Federation of Labour, July 20, 1994.
6. Davies, Ward and Beck: Barristers & Solicitors, "Outline of Proposal Affecting Laboratories and Specimen Collection Centres and the Government of Ontario re: Industry Cap and Related Matters," March 27, 1997.
7. OMA Section on Laboratory Medicine, Council Meeting minutes, September 20, 1996.
8. Robert K. Muir, OHA Chief Operating Officer, "Laboratory Service Funding Consultation," memo to OHA Member Institutions, August 18, 1998.
9. Leah Casselman, President, OPSEU, and Doug Health, Chair of OPSEU Medical Division, letter to Dawn Ogram, Director, Laboratory Services Restructuring Secretariat, September 24, 1998.
10. Chris Madill, OPSEU Staff, "Report of the Meeting [explaining the RFP process] of the Respondents in Hamilton," January 26, 1999.
11. THiiNC Health, "East 1 Regional Laboratory Services Plan: Ontario Regional Laboratory Service Planning," May 15, 2001.
12. "Laboratory Medicine Funding Framework Agreement Between: The Ontario Medical Association and Her Majesty Queen in Right of Ontario, as represented by the Minister of Health and Long-Term Care," March 30, 2005.
13. OMA Section of Laboratory Medicine, Minutes of the Section Council, Tuesday, February 3, 2004.
14. "The Toronto Hospital Signs Letter of Intent with MDS," *Labreport: News from the Toronto Hospital Laboratories,* 3(1), March, 1995.
15. David Wright, lawyer with Ryder Wright Blair and Doyle, "Timmins and District

Hospital – Partnership with GDML," letter to Jill Morgan, Job Security Officer, OPSEU, June 20, 1996.

16. "Agreement between the Ontario Association of Medical Laboratories ("OAML") and her Majesty the Queen in right for Ontario, represented by the Ministry of Health and Long-Term Care ("the Ministry)," March 17, 2003.

Chapter 5

The Winners — MDS, GDML and CML

The uncontested winners after forty years of the Ontario government's medical laboratory policy are three laboratory corporations, LifeLabs (formerly MDS), CML Healthcare Fund (CML) and Gamma-Dynacare Medical Laboratories (GDML). These three firms deliver about half the medical laboratory services in Ontario and operate profitably in five other provinces. Canadian public health care funds paid at least one billion dollars to these three companies in 2010, $650 million of which came from OHIP in Ontario. This is a conservative estimate. It does not include income from companies in which they are silent partners, nor does it include income from public organizations such as hospitals that contract with them for tests, management and other consulting services, nor does it include payments from other federal and provincial agencies and ministries, such as Indian Affairs, Corrections, Defence and workers' compensation programs.

These three corporations have a few things in common. All have their roots in small pathologist-owned laboratories that started in the 1960s. The physicians involved in founding these companies also worked in the public hospital laboratory system. The core source of their income through most of their corporate existence has been diagnostic laboratory services paid for out of public funds. This stable platform allowed them to expand into other private health care concerns which are rapidly increasing in cost undercutting the financial stability of public health care, including pharmaceuticals, diagnostic imaging and medical technologies. This funding allowed these corporations to become large multinational health care companies exporting private health care around the world.

All the companies have been consistently profitable; even in times of recession, yields to investors were above 8 percent with profit rates as high as 44 percent. The Canadian operations of these three multinationals have usually outperformed their U.S. counterparts, and the laboratory services components of these companies generally outperformed their other ventures. The strength of the laboratory services is probably due to the stability, lack of competition and long-term funding arrangements provided by universal health insurance and government regulation. Despite their nature as quasi public sector companies — they all rely primarily on public funds for their existence — the financial and operational information available on any of the three companies is limited.

LifeLabs/MDS

Of the big three, LifeLabs, formerly MDS, is the largest. It has also been studied the most. Many of the details in this summary are from Colleen Fuller's (1998; 1999) excellent history of MDS from 1970 to 1998.

MDS, short for Medical Data Sciences, was formed in 1969, "by five former employees of IBM's medical services division" (Fuller 1998: 246). It entered the clinical laboratory market by buying Toronto Medical Laboratories, a small chain of laboratories owned by Dr. Ley, the director of haematology at Toronto Western Hospital and a professor at the University of Toronto (Chemical Engineering Research 1969). MDS expanded across Canada, by acquiring smaller labs and buying into joint ventures with other local laboratory companies. During the 1970s, its profits were compounding at a rate of 18–20 percent per year, and 80 percent of its revenues came from public insurance fee-for-service payments (Fuller 1998). In 1997, diagnostic labs still produced one third of MDS's revenue and 40 percent of its profit (Austen 1997).

Starting in the 1990s, the company expanded into the U.S. diagnostic services market and branched out into other areas of health care. MDS's venture capital funds were used to start dozens of private health care companies, including acute care hospitals, pharmaceutical companies, orthopedic supply companies, home care agencies, nuclear medicine services, diagnostic technology services and a manufacturer of blood substitution products (Fuller 1999). By 1998, approximately half of the company's overall revenues were earned outside Canada, but the solid foundation was still laboratory services in Canada (Fuller 1999).

In all provinces where MDS operated in the 1990s, governments imposed some form of cost control. In the new millennium, MDS's strategy in Canada of joint ventures with hospitals and expansion in the government funded laboratory markets came to an end. From 2000 to 2005, MDS's stock values declined and it had a generally weak financial performance (Zehr 2005). Also, in 2005, MDS had revenues of $1.8 billion from medical supplies, drug development and returns on $1 billion in assets in health and life sciences venture capital funds, as well as laboratory services (MDS 2005). It was operating in twenty-seven countries and had 8,800 employees. Twenty-three percent of its revenues still came from general laboratory services but pharmaceuticals made up the largest share at 36 percent. Most important though is that by this time, MDS had become a global health care company, with 65 percent of its revenues coming from outside of Canada, and it wanted to focus on the more growth-oriented parts of its business.

In 2005, MDS joined Gamma-Dynacare in the U.S. tradition of questionable billing practices. MDS was found to have billed for two million claims that were covered or already paid for by U.S. health insurers (*Canadian Press* 2005).

The changing laboratory market, the changed nature of MDS and declining share value spelled the end of John Rogers, one of the founders of MDS, as president and CEO. In 2005, he was replaced by Stephen Defalco, a business consultant with experience in corporate restructuring. The hiring of Defalco as the CEO started a seismic shift in MDS. For the first time in its history none of the original MDS founders was at the helm and the company moved in a new direction. MDS Health Services Incorporated's 2005 annual report states: "Our new strategy is straightforward: focus on life sciences markets to drive growth and improve operating performance." In the company's opinion, the diagnostic laboratory business had matured and did not fit well with its new growth-oriented strategy, and investors agreed. With the expectation of more rapid growth, and more income for shareholders, partially financed by cash from the sale of its diagnostic services, when MDS announced that it was selling its medical laboratory division its stock value rose more than 12 percent (Prashad 2005). Once the decision to sell the diagnostic services had been made, the company focused on improving that division's profit margins. It instituted more cost-effective operating processes and a leaner, more accountable and more agile management structure. Overall, corporate staff was reduced by 36 percent; 700 positions, or 8 percent of the total workforce, were eliminated.

In 2007, Borealis Infrastructure Management, an investment arm of the Ontario Municipal Employees' Retirement Services pension fund, bought MDS's Canadian diagnostic services and changed its name to LifeLabs (Zehr 2006). The $1.3 billion that MDS received for its laboratory services was used to buy back shares, increasing MDS's profit per share, and to pay for MDS's purchase of Molecular Devices Corp. in California (Valorzi 2007). After MDS's diagnostic services division was sold, this Canadian company, built on public funds, was doing 95 percent of its business outside of Canada.

Borealis's mission is to invest in private companies that provide public services, often undercutting the jobs of the workers who pay into the pension fund that owns Borealis. While government-funded laboratory services do not have the growth potential that MDS wanted, they seemed a good fit with a pension fund and will probably provide a steady flow of income.

The pension fund management continued to operate LifeLabs as a business rather than an essential public service, hiring CEOs primarily for their private sector business credentials. In early 2009, Ida Goodreau, former president and CEO of Vancouver Coastal Health, one of British Columbia's largest health regions, was appointed CEO of LifeLabs. Before her job with the Coastal Health Authority, she had a long history in the pulp and paper industry. She left LifeLabs in December 2009 for personal reasons (Korstrom 2010). Goodreau was replaced by Jos Wintermans, LifeLabs' third president and CEO in as many years. Wintermans was another leader with extensive business experience outside of health care. He was a past CEO of Canadian Tire and of Sodisco-Howden Inc, a distributor of hardware products.

As well as its clinical laboratory business, LifeLabs supplies various services to government and private business that do not fall under medical insurance. By its own accounting, it is Canada's largest provider of specialty lab testing from early detection of cancer to DNA parentage testing. It continues to provide services to hospitals, including management, consulting, transportation, quality assurance and point-of-care testing. And it provides a wide range of professional health services to governments, industry and insurance companies, including occupational health and safety testing, drug testing and organizing clinical studies for new drugs (LifeLabs.ca).

In 2006, LifeLabs was reported to have 2,900 employees and revenues of

$335 million (Zehr 2006). It operates as LifeLabs in Ontario, British Columbia and Quebec. In Alberta it holds a majority interest in DynaLIFE. The company has a history of business partnerships, sometimes as a silent partner, and is probably a part owner, or even a majority owner, of a number of smaller labs in these and other provinces. There is very little public information on the operations of LifeLabs because it is privately held by Borealis.

Gamma-Dynacare Medical Laboratories (GDML)

Of Canada's three big laboratory companies, GDML is the most commercialized in the sense that it has been bought and sold by a series of investors and holding companies as an investment property. GDML's roots can also be traced back to private labs started by entrepreneurial pathologists in the 1960s, but it did not come together as a corporate entity until the 1990s. GDML is the result of the mergers of many smaller laboratories, with the core of its present structure emerging in the 1980s. The Latner family of Toronto, using money made from an overheated real estate market, set up Dynacare, a health care conglomerate that brought together Kopp Laboratories, which in 1968 was owned by a group of fourteen physicians, Kipling Medical Laboratories, which was founded before 1966, Quality Medical Laboratories, and other private health care operations, including nursing homes and home care services. Over the next decade, Dynacare's laboratory division incorporated Biochemistry Reference Laboratory, Douglas Laboratory Services, Elixir Medical Laboratories and Park-Med Laboratories before merging with Gamma North Peel Laboratory and Bio-Science Laboratory (Ontario) in 1997 to become GDML.

GDML further expanded by purchasing operations in the United States to become that country's sixth largest laboratory services company by 1998. The Latners sold the company to a Chicago-based venture capital firm in 1997. In 2002, Laboratory Corporation of America, LabCorp, the second largest U.S. laboratory service provider, purchased GDML for $480 million (US) and assumed $205 million worth of debt. At the time of the purchase, GDML had revenues of $402 million (*Hamilton Spectator* 2002). In 2010, LabCorp owned 85 percent of GDML. The 15 percent of GDML not owned by LabCorp was acquired by an unidentified partner in 2010.

LabCorp was interested in GDML partly because of its expertise in providing inpatient laboratory services (Harding 2002). GDML had made significant entrees into Canada's inpatient market at Sunnybrook in Toronto, the Ottawa regional hospitals and hospitals in Edmonton, Alberta. Eight years after its acquisition by LabCorp, all of these forays into inpatient services by GDML had ended.

In the last five years, GDML pursued its historical growth strategy of buying up existing independent laboratories. This has also been the preferred method of growth for its U.S. parent. In 2008, GDML purchased Manitoba's largest private laboratory, Central Medical Labs, and it now owns LDS laboratories in Quebec. In Saskatchewan, GDML is contracted by both the Saskatoon and the Regina Qu'Appelle Health Regions to run their specimen collections centres and specimen transfer services and to purchase their laboratory supplies. GDML owns 43.4 percent of Alberta's DynaLIFE, an investment valued at $57 million in 2009. GDML's consulting services were used by the province of New Brunswick in 2007 to evaluate a pathologist's work that was suspect.

Headquartered in Brampton, Ontario, GDML operates three laboratories in Ontario (Brampton, London and Ottawa), one in Montreal, one in Winnipeg and a network of more than 150 specimen collection centres nationwide. GDML employs more than 2,000 workers and has been recognized as one of the top 100 employers in the Toronto area. In 2007, operations in Ontario produced an income of $64 million for LabCorp on sales of $221 million, which is a profit of 29 percent from Canadian health care budgets. Whether these operations have continued to be as profitable is hard to tell because, after 2007, income from Ontario was consolidated into the overall reporting for the company making it difficult to track changes in Canada (LabCorp 2009). Regardless, with total revenues of $4.7 billion and an operating profit of $2 billion in 2009 LabCorp's Canadian operations are a small part of its concerns.

LabCorp's foreign ownership of GDML raises serious questions about sovereignty. Under the *Patriot Act*, the U.S. government can compel LabCorp to reveal personal medical information on any of its patients from any of its subsidiaries to U.S. intelligence agencies. LabCorp could be forced by U.S. law to break privacy laws that protect most Canadians. This potential serious breach of individual rights and Canadian law is compounded by provisions under the North American Free Trade Agreement (NAFTA) that could allow LabCorp to restrict our provincial governments' ability to enact health care policy for the benefit of Canadians. U.S. ownership of GDML raises the possibility that LabCorp could file for compensation for the loss of its investment if provincial governments decided to end their contractual relationship with GDML and use a non-profit organization to deliver the services. This threat of legal action by LabCorp raises the stakes for any government considering increasing non-profit provision of laboratory services and decreasing the role of GDML (Sack Goldblatt Mitchell 2008). And ownership by LabCorp comes with other baggage. In 1997, LabCorp paid $187 million in fines to the U.S. government for billing for millions of tests that were not needed for diagnosis or treatment: a practice we would prefer to keep out of our health care services (Perry 1996).

CML HealthCare Income Fund (CML)

Canadian Medical Laboratories (CML) was founded in 1969 in Simcoe, Ontario, by pathologist Dr. John Mull. Mull continued as the principal shareholder and head of the company into the new millennium. In 2004, Mull still owned 44 percent of the shares, though he has since stopped playing an active role in the company. CML was a privately held company until its first public offering of shares in 1996.

While a private company, it grew partly through the buying up of smaller labs; its most significant acquisition was the 1991 purchase of Cybermedix,

Ontario's second largest lab company. Unlike MDS and GDML, CML did not venture into inpatient laboratory operations and stayed focused on Ontario's community market. After going public, CML purchased Excel Bestview Medical Laboratories, Metro-Medical Labs and in 1999 the bankrupt Med-Chem for $105 million, doubling its laboratory operations.

CML broadened its health care interests in 2000 by making what it describes as a "low risk" entry into the drug development industry by founding a subsidiary, Cipher Pharmaceuticals (CML 2001). Established as a debt-free company with significant capital reserves, Cipher describes itself as an "innovative drug development company focused on commercializing novel formulations of successful, currently marketed molecules using advanced drug delivery technologies" (cipherpharma.com). What this corporate statement means is that Cipher is involved in the controversial practice of creating me-too drugs. These copycat drugs slightly alter the formulation or delivery mechanisms of already existing drugs and usually produce little in extra medical value. They are notorious as one of the main driving forces behind rapidly rising drugs costs (Goozner 2004). These drugs put pressure on provincial governments to buy the newer version, further stretching health care dollars, and often allow companies to apply for a new patent, delaying the manufacture of a cheaper generic drug.

Continuing a cautious and focused acquisition strategy, CML purchased DC Diagnosticare to expand its non-laboratory diagnostic services across Canada and into the United States. DC Diagnosticare provides a full range of imaging services including x-ray, MRI, CT, bone density, nuclear medicine and mammography. This CML subsidiary was one of the successful bidders to run private diagnostic centres in Ontario when the provincial government made its ill-fated attempt to privatize MRI and CT services in 2003. CML has continued its steady acquisition of diagnostic imaging services in the United States. In 2009, these U.S. operations accounted for 30 percent of revenues.

CML responded to the problems of growth versus stable income as MDS did by splitting its company, but the shareholders in CML retained ownership of both parts. In 2004, CML split off the CML Health Care Fund, an income trust created to take advantage of the "reliable and attractive investment yield," a yield provided by the public payer (CML HealthCare Inc. 2003). Income trusts are controversial due to their negative effects on tax revenues and their benefits for investors. In essence the income trust structure allows CML to take lucrative tax breaks, funded at the public's expense, and mix them with public health care dollars to create strong returns for private investors. CML plans to return to a corporate structure in 2011, when many of the tax benefits for income trusts will end.

At the same time that the CML income trust was created, Cipher Pharmaceuticals was made an independent company to provide shareholders with all the growth potential that exists in the prescription drug industry. Cipher had revenues of $3.2 million in 2009 and trades on the Toronto Stock Exchange. In 2004, it was reported that CML operated at substantially higher margins in Ontario than MDS (Zehr 2005), probably because its business was more focused on larger urban areas and centralized facilities. CML's Canadian operations also performed better than its U.S. holdings (Gibbs and El-Makkawy 2009). CML's annual operating profit margins are often in the range of 40 percent (Cole 2004) and yields to investors, even in times of recession, are over 8 percent.

In 2009, CML had 121 specimen collection centres in Ontario and one centralized laboratory in Mississauga. Eighty-five percent of its laboratory services income came from OHIP payments and the rest from selling tests to private-pay patients. Laboratory services provided 45 percent of the income trust's revenues. CML has become an international corporation with sales of $517 million (CML Healthcare 2009).

Chapter 6

Variations from Sea to Sea

Canadian federalism leaves the organization and delivery of health services to the provinces. However, the federal government's greater ability to raise money gives it power to negotiate national programs and standards for health care. This federal-provincial dynamic is evident in the delivery of laboratory services across Canada.

Canada's medical laboratory systems exhibit both a significant variety in evolution, funding and delivery, and important commonalties. A dominant factor in Canadian medical laboratory services is the continued centrality of non-profit facilities based in hospitals and public health laboratories. These facilities provide most inpatient services, emergency services, services to smaller communities, pathology testing, complex and labour-intensive testing and in six provinces most of the laboratory work for all patients. They are the backbone of this aspect of our medical system. This is largely due to the *Health Insurance and Diagnostic Services Act* of 1957, which tied federal funding to non-profit hospitals and mandated that hospitals provide laboratory services.

Six provinces, British Columbia to Quebec, use a mix of public and private laboratories for community patients. All but Quebec started out the same way, with public hospitals delivering inpatient care and some outpatient services and private laboratories being paid fee-for-service by medicare for community work, yet each has developed along a different path. The big divergences came in the mid-1990s when out-of-control laboratory spending, largely due to the private sector, clashed with funding cuts due to the neoliberal restructuring of the federal and provincial budgets.

Quebec has never made direct payments to private labs from public insurance. Quebec is the only province in which private payment for essential tests is possible, although the vast majority of community tests are publicly covered and processed in hospital laboratories. Ontario is the only province in which hospital laboratories have stopped processing specimens from community patients. Saskatchewan is the only province with a history of a vibrant private sector that has virtually stopped using for-profit laboratories to process specimens. The four Atlantic Provinces have no significant for-profit laboratory services.

LifeLabs, GDML and CML, the three corporations that dominate Canada's private laboratory services, started in Ontario and now operate in five other provinces. Only four provinces still use fee-for-service mechanisms to pay for corporate laboratory services and these all have hybridized systems. All provinces use some form of global budgeting or fixed-price contracts to fund most of their laboratories. Ontario has the greatest involvement of for-profit corporations, and

British Columbia, the second highest user of private services, has the highest per capita cost.

All provinces would like to have fully integrated laboratory information and production systems linked to all physicians. All currently have integration plans at least partially driven by the Canada Health Infoway, a federally funded agency with a $1.6 billion fund to increase the use of electronic health records. This program comes with the twist compared to the federal programs that built the non-profit laboratory network a half century earlier: most of the money is going to for-profit electronic medical records vendors. Most provinces have, at least, developed regional computerized laboratory links between hospitals with access for hospital staff. The private companies often have their own internal systems. Partly due to the existence of these competing systems, no province is close to meeting its broader integration goals.

Nova Scotia has recently won national praise for its rapid introduction of a province-wide system that creates the possibility for any doctor in the province to access any laboratory record. A major factor credited for this feat, unique among Canadian provinces, is "the single government run lab system, which greatly facilitated the process" (Chernos 2009). While it is still used by only a minority of family physicians, partially due to a lack of funding to support the conversion of their practices, the infrastructure is in place and can easily be added to.

Over the last five years, there has been a small move away from using for-profit laboratories. Continued strong support for public health care, tighter government funding and more regional health systems have forced health delivery organizations to adopt less expensive options than fee-for-service systems of payment. Simultaneously, private corporations have become less aggressive as restrictions on public funding have limited their growth potential. This happened in Saskatchewan when regional governments dropped the private laboratories as providers because of cost, and in Alberta some of the for-profit labs were nationalized. Nationally, as mentioned previously, MDS divested itself of its diagnostic laboratory division in 2007 because of limited growth potential.

Instead of increasing for-profit delivery, governments from coast to coast, limited by reduced revenue following extensive tax cuts, are restructuring the public non-profit laboratories along business lines. This has meant significant income opportunities for private consulting firms, for example, Corpus Sanchez, THiiNC Consulting and QSE Consulting, as well as for the three big lab companies. Public, non-profit laboratory systems have cut costs, reduced staff, speeded up work, down-skilled, centralized and introduced private business management styles, often to the detriment of smaller hospitals, patient access, staff recruitment and quality controls. These restructuring measures have not gone unchallenged. A successful resistance movement in Newfoundland and Labrador stopped the centralization of laboratory facilities that would have reduced service in Lewisporte and Flower's Cove (CBC Web News 2009).

Some of the restructuring creates potential openings for private corporations.

For example, the creation of discrete non-profit corporations, such as Diagnostic Services Manitoba, the Eastern Ontario Regional Laboratory Corporation and the Calgary Laboratory Services, to coordinate and provide inpatient laboratory services, especially if they involve stand-alone laboratory facilities, may improve service, but they also make it easier for a commercial operator to buy the discreet company or contract its management. Increased data integration could facilitate private laboratories' processing of some of the easier, less urgent inpatient work because the results would be readily available to hospital staff doctors. Regional data integration was a key component in privatizing most Edmonton hospital laboratory work in 1995 (Fagg et al. 1999).

Although heath care systems are changing at a rapid rate, it seems that laboratory services are changing more rapidly. The following summaries are not comprehensive reviews of each province's laboratory services. This would require a book for each province, updated yearly. These snapshots attempt to draw out information and connections between laboratory funding, ownership and delivery. Comprehensive government studies on laboratory services in Ontario, British Columbia and Saskatchewan, all in response to out-of-control costs and significant system dysfunction due to the presence of for-profit laboratories, have been a good source of information. Most other provinces have subsumed their laboratory services evaluations under larger health care restructuring, making access to data difficult. The problem is compounded when laboratory services and data are based in regional health authorities with little provincial coordination. The following summaries rely heavily on interviews with individuals active in their province's laboratory systems.

British Columbia

In the 1970s the BC government threatened sanctions against doctors who used the growing for-profit sector instead of hospitals for their laboratory work (*CMAJ* 1971). While this policy did not stop the development of vibrant for-profit laboratory corporations, it did lead to the creation of a system unique in Canada, in which hospitals are also paid fee-for-service from the medical services budget for processing community laboratory specimens.

Small private laboratories in British Columbia, as in Ontario, grew and consolidated after the introduction of universal medical insurance. By the early 1980s, BC Biomedical Services, Island Laboratory Services and Metropolitan (Metro-McNair) Laboratories emerged as the three main players.

BC Biomedical Services was founded by pathologist Dr. Coady in 1958 to provide services to hospitals in the lower mainland, an area of high population density. Its main laboratory is in Burnaby and it is now run by a consortium of forty-two pathologists. Multiple interlocking directorships between the pathologists involved in BC Biomedical and hospital laboratories have led to allegations of conflict of interest. It is claimed that easier, more profitable work is shunted from the hospital laboratories to BC Biomedical (Ohmert 2010, personal communication). This may explain why the Fraser Valley Health Region, where

Biomedical is heavily involved, has the highest percentage, 87 percent compared to 70 percent for the next highest region, of community laboratory work done in private laboratories (Bayne 2003).

Metro Laboratories was founded by another pathologist, Dr. Rix, in the 1960s. In the early 1980s it entered into a partnership with MDS to form MDS Metro, 75 percent owned by MDS, and now wholly owned by LifeLabs. It provides services throughout the province though it concentrates on the lower mainland. Island Medical Laboratory Services, the third largest regional laboratory, was also swallowed up MDS.

Two public studies of medical laboratories were conducted due to alarm over rising costs and utilization (Bayne 2003; British Columbia Ministry of Health 1993). British Columbia was found to have the highest per capita lab costs in Canada in 2006/07: $141 per person compared with a national average of $108. In part these high costs were due to the fact that both hospitals and private laboratories were paid fee-for-service for community laboratory services. As in other provinces, the cost of fee-for-service laboratory services had risen faster than the cost of inpatient laboratory services. In 2005, the private laboratories had profit margins estimated by laboratory specialists at 44 percent, and hospitals have advised their laboratories to increase their outpatient work as a revenue source.

British Columbia's experience argues against the level-playing-field between hospital and for-profit laboratories, an approach that has been suggested in Ontario as a way of putting the private laboratories out of business. The BC payment structure probably limited the development of private laboratory services (private labs deliver about 70 percent of the community work compared to 100 percent in Ontario), and it did put more money into the hands of hospitals. In 2001, hospitals earned about $80 million from community laboratory work (Bayne 2003). But it did not put the for-profit labs out of business.

An article praising BC Biomedical's working conditions noted that most staff work a thirty-five-hour weekday shift, indicating that most of the private laboratory facilities are not used during the evenings, nights and weekends (Sutherland 2004). Hospitals, due to the flow of inpatient work, usually have excess capacity, which when added to this private sector redundancy, probably contributed to British Columbia's high overall costs. As well as out-of-control costs, the system was extensively fragmented. In 2003, there were, according to the Bayne report, twenty-seven different laboratory information systems in the province.

In September 2003, after the publication of the Bayne report, fees paid for outpatient laboratory work were cut by 8 percent. They were cut a further 12 percent in April 2004. The financial blow from the fee reductions was partially offset, as MDS noted in its 2005 annual report, by moderate increases in volume due to population increases. Other changes were that the fee schedule is to be reviewed yearly by the Medical Service Commission in consultation with the BCMA. There is a utilization discount for the top thirty tests, which means that when the number of tests increases beyond certain thresholds the fees decrease, though the thresholds are increasing. And, the locations of specimen collection centres are now determined by a more open process.

Since the Bayne report, the rate of increase in outpatient laboratory expenditures has fallen from 44 percent over the four years 1997/98 to 2001/02, to 13 percent from 2004/05 to 2008/09. In 2008/09, $295 million was spent on outpatient laboratory services (British Columbia Ministry of Health Services 2010).

Bayne also proposed a regionally integrated model with one provider for all laboratory services, similar to the RFP model tried in Ontario, but it was scuttled by opposition from the private industry and the BCMA. Similar recommendations had been made before and rejected. A provincial laboratory coordination office set up in 2004 met with limited success and has since folded.

While there have been some changes, the basic structure of most of British Columbia's laboratory services remains the same. Inpatient services are funded through the global budgets of the regional health authorities, and both hospitals and private labs continue to be paid fee-for-service for outpatient services.

Alberta

The history of laboratories in Alberta is one of the more interesting and paradoxical. It has had some of the deepest incursions of for-profit laboratories into all corners of health care delivery yet Calgary's laboratory services were nationalized in 2006. Alberta, alone among the provinces with private laboratory services, has the distinction of having nearly all its medical laboratory technologists and assistants unionized.

As far back as the 1960s, Alberta had a significant number of private laboratories run by local pathologists. They were parochial and took a strong anti-commercial stand in 1970 against a large U.S. pharmaceutical company, Smith, Kline and French from Philadelphia, that wanted to buy one of the larger for-profit laboratories (Bell 1970). By the 1990s, most community laboratory services in the two large urban areas, Calgary and Edmonton, were provided by for-profit corporations on a fee-for-service basis, and hospitals provided inpatient services out of their global budgets. In 1994, hospital and for-profit laboratories split the $244 million spent on medical laboratory services evenly (Fagg et al. 1999). Kasper Laboratories, started by the pathologist Dr. T.A. Kasper, was then Alberta's largest for-profit laboratory. In southern Alberta, outside of Calgary, most services were provided through hospital-based regional structures.

In the mid-1990s, working in conjunction with the Alberta Medical Association, the provincial government set up an elaborate framework that facilitated the expansion and regulation of for-profit health care companies (Plain 2000). To control costs and facilitate privatization, seventeen regional health authorities (RHA) were established to run most health services in their areas. Each RHA was given a budget for laboratory services that equalled 53 percent of the payments previously made to private laboratories and 75 percent of the public sector payment. This arrangement ended fee-for-service payments to pathologists (Fagg et al. 1999). After a failed attempt to have private companies submit an RFP to provide laboratory services in each region, the Klein government cajoled the major private laboratories in Edmonton and Calgary into forming consortiums to run all of the laboratory services. The Health Sciences Association of Alberta, the laboratory workers' union, argued for a chance to bid on delivering the laboratory services, but the suggestion was rejected by the provincial government (Ballerman 2010, personal communication).

In the Capital Health Region, around Edmonton, three local private sector labs joined forces with Gamma-Dynacare and MDS (MDS was a silent partner) to form Dynacare-Kasper Medical Laboratories (DKML). DKML was given the contract for all laboratory services except for services for inpatients in the University of Alberta Hospital, which stayed in the public sector. Other hospital laboratories were turned into rapid response laboratories and managed by DKML. DKML continued to process the community work in their stand-alone laboratories. The regionalization in Edmonton cut laboratory expenses by 40 percent, eliminated 357 jobs in the public sector, added 80 jobs to the private sector, cut the number of SCCs from 129 to 27 and instituted a regional laboratory information system connecting all laboratories and SCCs (Fagg et al. 1999).

The Calgary Regional Health Authority (CRHA) set up a public-private partnership with Kasper, MDS and its own company, Calgary Laboratory Services (CLS), to provide all the services in the region. The CRHA held a 50 percent interest in the new company. CLS has a separate laboratory facility that processes most of the community and inpatient specimens, and the hospitals have rapid response laboratories (Swaine 2010, personal communication). As in Edmonton, there was a significant reduction in collection centres as funding was cut (Coopers & Lybrand 1997). In 2009, CLS ran eighteen patient care centres, their name for community specimen collection centres.

In 2005, there was a significant move to bring parts of Alberta's laboratory services back into the public sector. In the Capital Health Region, around Edmonton, hospital inpatient services were brought back under hospital management. DKML continued to provide community laboratory services and own and run the laboratory in the Fort McMurray Hospital (Ballerman 2010, personal communication). LifeLabs then bought out all the local interests in DKML and, in partnership with Gamma-Dynacare, now runs this corporation under the name DynaLIFE.

In 2006, when MDS decided to sell its diagnostic laboratory division, the CRHA paid it $21 million for its 26 percent interest in CLS and bought out Kasper-Dynacare's share to gain complete control of CLS, effectively creating a fully integrated public laboratory system in Calgary. CLS continues as a stand-alone non-profit corporation that owns the laboratory equipment, hires the staff, rents space in hospitals and runs its own facility and specimen collection to deliver all the laboratory services in the Calgary region.

In 2008, Alberta centralized all health services under the Alberta Health Services Board (AHS). It owns all the hospital laboratories and Calgary

Laboratory Services, and it contracts DynaLIFE to provide community services in the Edmonton area and all laboratory services in the northeastern region. CLS is financed through a global budget from the Alberta Health Services. DynaLIFE is paid an administrative fee and a fee for each test. To help control utilization there is a volume discount. Over a certain number of tests the price paid per test decreases. There is no hard cap on payments. DynaLIFE's contract runs out in 2016 (Hofer 2010, personal communication). Except for a contract with one other small private laboratory in Medicine Hat all other inpatient and community laboratory services are delivered through the AHS hospitals or in doctors' clinics.

AHS's goal is a province-wide integration of all laboratory services to reduce duplication and improve coordination of services. As well as acute care and community services, the AHS laboratory services runs the cancer laboratories and public health services. AHS's first step to provincial integration was to consolidate pap smears into two facilities, DynaLIFE's central laboratory in Edmonton and the Calgary Regional Laboratory. Pathologists and community organizations have criticized the move, saying it will weaken hospitals and hurt the training of new laboratory specialists, a professional group already in short supply (Sinnema 2010). The move of more public sector work to the for-profit DynaLIFE raises the spectre of conflict of interest. Jennifer Rice, a former medical director of DynaLIFE, headed the transition team that made this recommendation and Charlotte Robb, a former DynaLIFE CEO, was the first CEO of the new Alberta Health Services Board (Lang 2009).

Saskatchewan

In the early 1990s, Saskatchewan had a fragmented laboratory system with significant overcapacity, duplication and rapidly rising costs. Along with the hospital system and a provincial laboratory, which still performed community laboratory work as well as reference work and public health testing, there were eight for-profit laboratories. These private labs provided 21 percent of the province's haematology services, 27 percent of the biochemistry work and 30 percent of microbiology assays and accounted for 29 percent of the costs. Between 1988 and 1992, private sector laboratory costs grew 49 percent compared to 33 percent for hospital laboratory costs (Kilshaw et al. 1992).

An internal government report found that the cost of using hospital laboratories, depending on whether a marginal cost or a unit cost approach was taken, was 30 percent and 70 percent respectively of what for-profit laboratories charged for the same service (Saskatchewan Health 1991). The province's negative experience with private laboratories is one of the factors behind the NDP government's passage of the *Health Facilities Licensing Act* of 1996, which made it virtually impossible for private health care facilities to thrive in the province (MacIntosh and Ducie 2009).

Following the recommendations of the Kilshaw review, conducted for the Ministry of Health in 1992, the recently established health districts were made responsible for the delivery of most laboratory services. Each district was given a laboratory budget roughly equivalent to the sum of the previous fee-for-service payments and hospital grant funding for diagnostic laboratory services.

Alone among the provinces with a publicly funded for-profit sector, Saskatchewan stopped processing specimens in commercial laboratories after the 1990s budget crunch. A number of factors led to this result. In 1991, MDS owned one of the largest private laboratories in the province and approached the NDP, which was expected to soon form the government, with a plan to use its company to deliver the province's laboratory services. The unions, concerned that the NDP might have made a deal to privatize the laboratories, mounted a campaign focusing on the higher costs of private laboratories (Smillie 2010, personal communication). There was also pressure from some of the newly elected NDP members of the Legislative Assembly to move away from private providers. The unpopular closing of many small rural hospitals also created a need for the NDP to be seen to be supporters of public health care. The government was also looking for ways to save money in its health care budget to reduce its provincial deficit, and there was a general understanding that one area where money could be saved was in laboratory services (Simard 2010, personal communication).

The result of these influences was "a very clear intention" on the part of the government and the bureaucracy to integrate services, including diagnostics, in the public sphere through the newly formed health districts (Perrins 2010, personal communication). In 1996, MDS lost its contract to provide laboratory services in Regina. The work was brought back into the hospital system. The Prince Albert District saved 40 percent of its laboratory costs when it brought all laboratory work back into the public hospitals after the regionalization of services (Commission on the Future of Health Care in Canada 2002). Since the government did not ban the use of for-profit services, MDS, through its Saskatchewan-based company Medical Arts Laboratory, was retained to manage the restructuring of the Saskatoon Region's laboratories, which resulted in dozens of employees being laid off and having to reapply for their positions (Parker 1996). Saskatoon has since moved the management of all laboratory processing back into the public sphere.

Currently, almost all laboratory work in Saskatchewan is processed in public facilities though the two largest health regions, Regina and Saskatoon, contract out their specimen collection, supply procurement and specimen transportation. Gamma-Dynacare won this contract away from MDS in 2004 (Rempel 2004) and was paid $5.5 million in 2009 for its services. MDS had to pay its workers $2 million in severance charges when it lost the contract (Erwin 2004).

Physicians perform a limited number of tests in their clinics, but the amount paid for these services has dropped from $1.7 million in 2005/06 to $1.4 million in 2008/09 (Saskatchewan Health 2009). Gamma-Dynacare performs a small number of tests, like pregnancy testing and urinalysis, at some of its specimen collection centres under contract with the health authorities.

Manitoba

Manitoba also developed two separate laboratory streams: fee-for-service private laboratories and non-profit laboratories' services covered under global hospital budgets or directly from the public health budget. Concerns in the 1990s about the system's fragmentation, cost and staffing brought about two major changes. In 1995, a hard cap was placed on fee-for-service payments to private laboratories. The funding cap initially cut total payments to the sector by over 20 percent, with the expectation that the same number of tests would be conducted (Coopers & Lybrand 1997). The caps have continued through a series of negotiated agreements between the Ministry of Health and Doctors Manitoba, formerly the Manitoba Medical Association. The current agreement, which both the Ministry and Doctors Manitoba declined to make public, will expire in 2011. The 2010 cap is $29 million divided between eight laboratory companies based on their percentage of billed services (Jamieson 2010, personal communication). From 2001 to 2010, payments to the for-profit laboratories increased by approximately 8.8 percent. Under pressure from funding restrictions, private laboratories have consolidated over the last two decades. In 2008, Gamma-Dynacare purchased the largest private company, Central Medical Laboratories.

The second major change in the late 1990s was a move to centralize and possibly privatize hospital laboratory services, especially in rural Manitoba. This plan changed with the election of an NDP government in 1999. Diagnostic Services of Manitoba (DSM), an arms-length, non-profit, province-wide organization, was created to restructure hospital laboratories. DSM owns all of the laboratory equipment, hires the staff and operates all the facilities. It rents the laboratory space from the regional health authorities (RHA). While the rent is a paper transaction, it is part of an effort to reflect the true costs of doing business for comparison to the for-profit sector. The board of directors of DSM includes representatives from the RHAs and laboratory workers' unions.

Initially, DSM was to charge the health authorities on a fee-for-service basis for tests ordered. This was found to be unworkable because some of the smaller hospitals order very few tests yet need to have a laboratory in their community to complement other medical services. The fee-for-service revenue would not have come close to reflecting the true costs of maintaining these small laboratories. DSM changed to billing each RHA for the costs of staff, supplies and equipment used at laboratory facilities in their regions. The other main change from DSM's original mandate is that, other than in Winnipeg and Brandon, DSM now also delivers diagnostic imaging services. Since many of the smaller hospitals use the same technologists to staff the imaging services and the laboratory, this was a logical step (Dalton 2010, personal communication).

DSM collects and processes the community laboratory work outside of Brandon and Winnipeg. In Brandon and Winnipeg community patients go to private labs. DSM has actively discouraged community patients from coming to its facilities in these centres because the RHAs receive no extra funding for these patients. Ninety-five percent of DSM's funding comes from the RHAs, which operate on global budgets from the province.

In both Winnipeg and Brandon, DSM's facilities are linked by databases that are accessible to hospital physicians in the region. There are no computer links with the private labs. This has likely led to an increase in redundant testing. When community patients are admitted, the hospital staff like to have current laboratory data in the computer so they may reorder tests that have been recently done in a private lab and are probably not needed (Dalton 2010, personal communication).

Also receiving fee-for-service payments from Manitoba's provincial health insurance is an extensive network of small laboratories run by family doctors and primary care clinics. There were 769 of these in the mid-1990s (Coopers & Lybrand 1997). No information on the current number of doctors involved or the cost was provided the Manitoba government.

Quebec

Of the more populous provinces, Quebec has taken a unique path. With the introduction of medicare, the government mandated that medical laboratory tests would only be covered if they were performed in a public facility, usually a hospital. This policy continues today. It would take more comprehensive research to determine exactly why Quebec took this approach to diagnostic services, but Malcolm Taylor's (1978) description of the forces involved in the introduction of medicare in Quebec provides some clues. Quebec had relatively weak private insurance programs before medicare, which would have meant that there was less funding available for private laboratory services than in other provinces. The medical profession was more fractured than in other provinces, and there was a strong popular campaign for state medical services and for limiting the power of specialists, including pathologists. These factors coupled with the development of non-profit community health care centres, the CLSCs, as the centre of primary care, probably left little room for the development of private, publicly funded medical services such as commercial laboratories.

Also unique in Quebec, for-profit laboratories operate completely outside medicare and provide medically necessary tests to patients who pay privately, either personally or through private insurance. The roots of this parallel private system are also in the struggles around the introduction of medicare. A bitter strike by specialists won them the right to opt out of medicare, but their patients, unlike in Ontario, were not allowed public compensation for privately purchased services.

In many ways Quebec's private laboratory services are complementary to the system of private imaging facilities and surgeries that exist in Montreal, a city that has been described as the "Mecca of private health care in Canada" (Derfel 2005a). There are no readily available statistics to show how much laboratory work is processed in the private laboratories, or whether and how these laboratories are tied to the other private health care facilities in the Montreal region, though they are often linked on company websites. One estimate is that private laboratories accounted for 4.5 percent of Quebec's laboratory services in 1990 (Kilshaw et al. 1992), and another claims their income was over $30 million in 2005 (Derfel 2005b).

Quebec has the lowest per capita laboratory expenses in Canada (see Table 7-1 in the next chapter). Although Quebec is excluded from reporting by the Canadian Institute for Health Information and does not use the same MIS database as the other provinces, Quebec's Ministry of Health and Social Services reports that it spent $466 million on 119 public sector medical laboratories and 350 SCCs in 2007: a greater number of SCCs per capita than in Ontario (Levert 2010, personal communication; Ministère de la Santé 2008).

All the major national laboratory chains now provide services in Quebec, mostly in the Montreal area. In 2005, Gamma-Dynacare bought out LDS Diagnostic Services, a Quebec-based company that had been in business since 1968. LDS's revenue increased 50 percent in 1998. Part of the increase came from a business strategy in which the company sets up collection stations near overcrowded hospitals and waits for frustrated patients with money or insurance to come across the street for their blood tests (Diekmeyer 2003). While these for-profit labs may not relieve pressure on the system, they help relieve pressure on the government by providing an option for financially secure patients. This strategy would have been particularly successful in 1998, when hospitals were suffering from cuts in federal transfer payments.

As well as the major chains, Quebec has private independent laboratory companies, for example, Biron Laboratories and Curalab. Some of Quebec's private laboratories increased their income by advertising themselves as full-service labs, charging patients full cost for a test, then taking the sample (without the patient's knowledge) to a public hospital and having it processed at a fraction of what the patient paid (Marriot 1993). It is also alleged that the private laboratories offer kickbacks to doctors for ordering superfluous tests (Derfel 2005b).

Quebec has recently been reorganized into ninety-five health and social services centres that integrate family doctors, hospitals, long-term care facilities, many community health and social services and public laboratory services. One advantage of limiting the development of private laboratories, or for that matter, other private networks, is that it is relatively easy to integrate services structurally when they are all already administered publicly. New initiatives, such as the 2005 group practice clinics in the Montreal region, are easily linked to public laboratory facilities. All the samples from these new clinics are processed in hospital laboratories. Similarly, all of the hospitals and the family group medical practices in the Saguenay-Lac St. Jean region are linked (Harvey 2010, personal communication). These initiatives are coordinated and paid for under the regional health authority's budget.

In contrast, when Ontario introduced the family health networks, similar to the Montreal clinics, the government stipulated that their laboratory work go to a private laboratory. The funding cap for laboratories was increased to accommodate the increase in work sent their way. Ontario's arrangement sustains a system with minimal integration and higher costs.

In response to the 2005 Supreme Court ruling allowing private insurance for some essential medical procedures in Quebec under specific conditions, the "Chaoulli decision," the Quebec government passed Bill 33, which permits private laboratories in Quebec to gain access to public money by processing work under contract with some hospitals (Prémont 2010, personal communication). Private facilities also receive a public subsidy in the form of tax breaks for residents who pay for private laboratory services or purchase private insurance.

New Brunswick

Laboratory services in New Brunswick are organized under two regional health authorities (RHAs) and funded out of their global budgets. There are no for-profit laboratories in this province. Each hospital operates a laboratory service with its own operating procedures and database. The government is spearheading a province-wide laboratory data integration initiative (Clarke 2010, personal communication). The RHAs run community collection centres as part of the public service.

There are also private phlebotomy companies, which, for a fee, take your sample, usually blood, and deliver it to the hospital laboratory. There is no provincial regulation of this service, but the RHAs require that such services use the hospital's collection equipment (blood tubes) and patient identification systems (Steeves 2010, personal communication).

In the mid-1990s, Gamma-Dynacare, MDS and consultants KPMG explored opening private laboratories in New Brunswick, but resistance in the public sector stopped these initiatives (Waldie 1996; Schneider 2010, personal communication). The province did contract Gamma-Dynacare in 2007 to do a retrospective review of 21,000 pathology cases that may have been read incorrectly. Gamma-Dynacare almost certainly used pathologists that were cross-employed in non-profit facilities, since most complicated pathology work in Canada is done in hospitals, indicating that the work could have been done by any number of public sector institutions, a move that would have strengthened Canada's non-profit laboratory services rather than siphoning money off into a for-profit laboratory.

Nova Scotia

All laboratory work in Nova Scotia is done in public hospitals; there are no private laboratories. Under the Capital District Health Authority (CDHA), the largest health region, there are eight processing laboratories and sixteen public specimen collection centres. Inpatients account for 23.8 percent of the work, 63.4 percent is for outpatients and community patients, and 12.8 percent comes from referrals from other health districts, the province's maternity and children's hospital, the IWK Health Centre, and other provinces (O'Brian 2010, personal communication).

Nova Scotia's laboratory services are organized by the district health authorities and funded through their global budgets. In line with recommendations from a review of the health care system done at a cost of $1.9 million by private consultants Corpus Sanchez (Buott 2010, personal communication), the province is setting up provincial systems for cancer testing and other programs as a start to consolidating laboratories provincially (Corpus Sanchez 2007).

The province held serious discussions with MDS in the 1990s (Waldie 1996), but the introduction of for-profit corporations "proved to be so complicated and expensive" that this option was not pursued (Crocker 2010, personal communication). While there are no private labs, there is a booming industry in private phlebotomy services involving "hundreds of companies," most of which are very small (O'Brian 2010, personal communication). Private phlebotomy companies usually charge $10–25 to take blood, which can be done in a person's home, at the top end of the fee scale, and in some pharmacies and doctors' offices. This is an unregulated industry; anyone can take someone's blood and bring it into a hospital for processing. To try to maintain quality, the CDHA has the private companies sign a contract agreeing that they will meet certain standards for transportation of the samples, timeliness, labelling and will provide the appropriate requisitions, or the samples will be rejected by the hospital laboratory and the doctor notified.

Under the Medical Services Insurance in Nova Scotia, doctors receive no extra money for taking or processing laboratory specimens, even urinalysis. Having a private phlebotomist use their facilities provides extra income for doctors and pharmacies (often a percentage of the income from taking the samples) (O'Brian 2010, personal communication). A patient relations officer at Doctors Nova Scotia, the professional organization, does not consider it a conflict of interest for a doctor to receive money from one of these services: "it is the patients' choice" (Mallam 2010, personal communication).

These private phlebotomy services increase access for some patients but create a two-tier system for an essential medical service, which is especially harmful to those who are sicker and require more blood work. These patients are forced to pay significant extra fees, possibly hundreds or thousands of dollars a year, or use a less convenient service. The community specimen collection centres set up by the CDHA were well received by the public, but there are "health resource challenges" that are preventing more from being established (O'Brian 2010, personal communication).

Prince Edward Island

At the time of writing, P.E.I. was reorganizing its health care system for the fourth time in fifteen years, joining most other provinces in an ongoing destabilization of their public health systems. Based on recommendations from international health consultants Corpus Sanchez (2008), the government is moving to a province-wide integration of its laboratory services. These will be organized under the new Health P.E.I., the health authority set up in 2010 to run an integrated island-wide health system. Corpus Sanchez also recommended increasing the number of outpatient collection centres and using point-of-care testing.

Until the changes come into effect, all laboratory work in P.E.I., including community work, is done in the province's seven hospitals. Laboratory services are organized around the two main referral hospitals, Queen Elizabeth Hospital (QEH) and Prince County Hospital. At QEH about 15 percent of the volume is inpatients, 15 percent is outpatients and 70 percent is community work. More esoteric lab work that has to be done off-island is usually sent to the Hospital-In-Common Laboratories in Ontario for processing. Laboratory results are centralized in one database and available by computer to all hospital doctors. There is no large-scale access to this database by community doctors.

Prince Edward Island has no private laboratories. Dave Schneider, laboratory manager at QEH, says that private labs have shown an interest in setting up in P.E.I. but that, "the volume of service was not large enough for them to really push for it" (2010, personal communication).

Newfoundland and Labrador

Most clinical laboratory work in Newfoundland and Labrador is processed in public hospitals or the provincial laboratory. Some point-of-care testing and simple lab work is done in rural and remote health clinics. All laboratory services, except the provincially run public health laboratory, are covered by the global budgets of the four regional health authorities (RHAs). Currently the regions are trying to centralize their services. This has met with significant opposition, and the Eastern Health Region's recent attempts to close laboratory facilities in Lewisporte and Flowers Cove were stopped.

Newfoundland and Labrador, like the other Atlantic Provinces, has no for-profit laboratories. Regulations under the *Medical Care Insurance Act* would permit the establishment of independent laboratories outside of hospitals, but this has not happened. The 1997 provincial budget documents raised the possibility that to save money medical laboratory services would be turned over to the private sector, but a negative public "backlash" forced the government to abandon the idea. Also for-profit laboratories, as other for-profit health services, have not been very interested in Newfoundland and Labrador because there is "no market here for companies to make huge profits" due to the small population with relatively complicated health needs, which do not lend themselves to simple profitable health services. There are small private phlebotomy services in St. John's that collect blood for a fee in people's homes (Connors 2010, personal communication). There are no proposals to establish private laboratories in Newfoundland, and such a development would raise governmental concerns because it would draw personnel from an already short-staffed public system (Collins 2010, personal communication).

Chapter 7

Cost and Integration

In 1977, Dennis Timbrell, Ontario's minister of health, told the OMA executive: "It is in the public interest that laboratory work, all of which is paid from public funds, be done at the lowest cost facility ... there is only one customer [the government]."[1] This insight goes to the heart of one of the central and more rancorous debates on medical laboratories: which costs more, hospitals or private facilities?

Claims of cost-effectiveness have a strong rhetorical appeal and have been central to laboratory policy discussions for the last fifty years. One proposed explanation of why for-profit corporations have done reasonably well in Ontario and the western provinces is that they have provided a more cost-effective medical laboratory service. This is the argument made by the commercial industry and supporters of increasing the role of for-profits in health care.

A significant part of the reason for the emotion in the cost debate is the high stakes involved. Total medical laboratory services account for over $4 billion of provincial health care budgets. Corporations are anxious to benefit from access to these public health care dollars. The public, on the other hand, benefits from the most effective use of these resources.

The political left has often dismissed calls for cost control as rhetoric to pressure for allowing more market forces into our public services or as a tool used to cut services. While this is certainly true, the efficient use of resources, represented by the surrogate indicator *cost*, is important. Leys (2001: 222) argues: "Progressive democrats need to be concerned with raising productivity in public services, as much as (or more than) market fundamentalists." Various indicators of improved productivity, such as whether the service fulfils its purpose from the point of view of the public, are used, but cost is very much part of the equation.

Seriously considering costs respects the fact that choices have to be made about how we use resources. In the current context, the argument that if profit-taking were removed, there would be sufficient resources to meet all the population's needs, is no longer plausible. There will still be conflicts over resources between health care, environmental clean-up, good housing, adequate incomes, a secure food supply and a variety of other pressing needs. Using resources to maximum benefit will make it possible to better address all of these. This reality is heightened by the increasing pressure placed on public policy by environmental degradation and global inequality. Any solution that aims for greater social justice needs to acknowledge, for example, that Canadians, on a per capita basis, use 300 times as much health care as do citizens of Mozambique.

When deciding how much to pay for laboratory services, it is not enough to say that the preferred choice is the one that leads to the lowest cost. Not providing publicly funded services would achieve that goal. Health care policies, includ-ing policies governing laboratory services, in a democratic and humane society need to consider issues of equity, fair compensation and security for workers, quality, access and public involvement. And all of these have costs associated with them. It is naive to think that there are no trade-offs, which is why wasting public money on for-profit solutions is ethically wrong when it comes to the delivery of an essential public service.

Timbrell's comments also point to one of the main conundrums for the for-profit laboratories. To make handsome profits from the delivery of health care, they need access to large sums of public money, and yet, from the perspective of the government, markedly so in neoliberal times, cost control and reduction of the state are hallmarks of good government and essential for increasing the power of the market and private profit. It was an issue for Ontario's Conservatives long before the Washington Consensus pushed reducing the size of the state onto the political agenda

This chapter looks at the impact of for-profit corporations on costs. Although a number of factors make it difficult to compare the costs, the weight of evidence and basic logic argue strongly that the use of for-profit laboratories increases health care costs. This conclusion is supported by the existence in Ontario of a natural experiment that goes to the heart of the debate. Many public, non-profit programs have provided the same community laboratory service as the com-mercial sector for decades at a fraction of the cost.

The Cost Argument for Non-Profit Laboratories

The logic of the argument for using the public sector, hospitals and public health laboratories as the main providers of community services is straightforward. Hospitals need on-site laboratory services in order to promptly meet the needs arising from emergency and inpatient care. This is recognized in Regulation 523, Section 33(1) of Ontario's *Public Hospitals Act*: "A hospital shall be equipped with a clinical laboratory with facilities and staff able to make routine investiga-tions necessary for the treatment of patients in the hospitals."

Hospitals need laboratories with the capacity to satisfy their daytime inpa-tient requirements. For most hospitals this means significant unused capacity and often underutilized staff in the evening and at night. Community laboratory work could be done in hospitals, with equipment that has already been paid for with public money, at times when the laboratory is not being used, in buildings that are already heated and maintained. The cost of processing this extra work becomes the marginal costs of extra staff, more reagents, and wear and tear on the machines and buildings. Increasing volumes in hospitals improves cost ef-ficiency; "because laboratories have relatively high fixed expenses, a reduced volume substantially increases unit costs" (Brenblum 1998). As well as increas-ing the efficiency of hospital laboratories, moving work out of a relatively more expensive fee-for-service environment and into the public sector will drive costs down farther.

The workflow in hospitals meshes nicely with the workflow in the community, where most specimens are collected during the day to be processed in the evening so that results are available the next day. The HICL achieved this level of integration in many communities where it collected community specimens and used hospital laboratories for processing.

The Private Sector Unit-Cost Approach

Not surprisingly, the above method of determining cost is not the one advocated by the private laboratory industry. The for-profit sector wants to compare the discrete unit costs of providing a test in a for-profit laboratory to the cost of performing the same test in a hospital, as if hospitals were just set up to provide laboratory services. There are a couple of daunting problems with the unit-cost comparison method.

Trying to compare hospital labs to private labs has confounded analysts for decades because of the differences between the two sites. Hospitals need to provide stat services, are usually more automated, do more esoteric and reference work and provide a greater percentage of labour intensive pathology, cytology and microbiology tests, and the hospital system provides services to many small and marginalized communities, which carries an inherently higher cost. Private laboratories need to pay their shareholders and run a system of collection centres. To complicate matters further, the sectors use different workload measures.

A second more fatal problem is that unit-cost comparison doesn't address the actual situation in Canada. For essential health services, there is only one payer, the government, and a hospital system is already in place. From the point of view of the public payer, the abstracted unit cost is not the main concern. What is relevant is the total cost to the system of providing the service. A senior Ontario Ministry of Health official in 1978 stated the position clearly: "There is a wide measure of agreement within the Ministry that hospitals should be funded on an incremental cost basis for the use of spare capacity for provision of out-patient laboratory services to the community."[2]

This is basic economics, and the provincial government in Ontario was recently reminded of this fact in a report on the last community non-profit providers in the province: "Automation and operating synergies enable incremental test volumes to be accommodated at low marginal costs" (RPO Management Consultants 2008: 78). The self-serving for-profit demand for definitive unit cost comparisons and dismissal of the marginal-cost approach is also disingenuous. The concept of marginal cost is common in business transactions; for example, increasing the quantity of an order usually reduces the per-unit cost. Also, the for-profit corporations adapted well to Ontario's and British Columbia's utilization discounts, as the number of tests goes up, the fee-for-service goes down, indicating that their marginal costs are still below the reduced fee-for-service rate.

Excess Capacity

The ability of hospitals to meet community demand is commonly accepted. In 1994, the head of the Ontario Hospital Association, commented: "There is massive reserve capacity in the hospital laboratories… a fully staffed evening shift could absorb the private laboratories' workload without difficulty" (Ontario Hospital Association 1994). This is most clearly the case for the more automated services such as hematology and chemistry, with many analyzers being idle for the better part of a twenty-four hour period. In 2010, Dr. Dalton, CEO of Diagnostic Services Manitoba, in a personal communication, agreed that the hospitals could handle the volume of the community work currently processed in the private laboratories on existing automated equipment. The RPO study (2008) of Ontario's pilot projects reported that most hospitals were able to process their community's laboratory work in less than four hours per day.

The consultants also identified excess capacity in Ontario's private sector (RPO 2008), which is mirrored by reports that BC Biomedical operates its main lab primarily on thirty-five hours per week, daytime shifts. Excess capacity in either system is primarily paid for with public funds and, except for the redundancy necessary to accommodate fluctuations in demand, is a waste.

Integration would lower unit costs. Savings realized through integration in the public system are savings to the Ministry, which means money available to be spent on other health care needs. Greater efficiencies in the private sector mean that "commercial laboratories can either reinvest savings in the business or pay them out to shareholders" (RPO 2008: 76).

The Evidence

Saving Money with Hospital Laboratories

The most compelling evidence that using hospitals to process community laboratory work saves money comes from two programs in Ontario: the Hospitals In-Common Laboratory (HICL) and the Hamilton Health Sciences Laboratory Program (HHSLP).

For thirty years the HICL provided community laboratory services for fee-for-service rates that were 75 percent of the rate paid to the commercial laboratories. At times this rate dropped to 66 percent of the commercial rate. These savings to the public system are understated. The HICL paid the hospitals for the tests processed in their labs, thereby injecting money back into the public laboratory system. A 2008 study of Ontario's pilot projects, most involving the HICL, found that they performed work for $22 per community patient, while the for-profit laboratories cost $33 (RPO 2008).

Published cost comparisons for 1990–91 indicate that the HHSLP's costs were 26.4 percent less than the cost would have been if a for-profit laboratory had performed the same work, a saving of $11 million to the system on the volume of community work done in Hamilton area hospitals (McQueen and Bailey 1993a, 1993b). Both the HICL and HHSLP ran a network of community specimen collection centres, provided in-home pickup and service to nursing home residents. At one point the HICL opened a collection centre in a drug store.

Both the HICL and HHSLP show that the use of hospitals to process community laboratory specimens can provide a long-term, stable, accessible, flexible and less costly service than using for-profit corporations. They provide the strongest evidence in favour of using hospital laboratories to process community laboratory work or, in the negative, against the proposal that there is a financial benefit to be gained from using for-profit laboratory corporations.

Marginal Cost

One study tried to calculate the marginal cost of bringing all the community laboratory testing into the hospital labs. The Ministry of Health in Saskatchewan undertook a calculation in 1992 and found that all the community tests could be done in public laboratories at 30 percent of the cost of using corporate labs. This cost determination is based on the extra staff, reagents, material and overhead needed to keep the hospital laboratories open long enough to process the community tests (Saskatchewan Health 1991).

Per Capita Cost

Another approach to studying cost is to examine how much governments pay per individual in the population served to deliver laboratory services, the per capita cost. THiiNC consultants prepared such figures for Lillian Bayne's review of laboratory services in British Columbia. The figures show that per capita laboratory expenditures were highest in the five provinces with active private laboratory corporations and lowest in those with no for-profit involvement (see Table 7-10). A similar finding can be made from the 1990/91 per capita cost comparisons done for Ontario's Laboratory Services Review.

Per capita comparisons using 2007 data revealed a similar pattern. Quebec's per capita expenses are the outlier in this table. They are both substantially less than the other provinces and the only province where per capita costs decreased in real dollars from 1991 to 2007. CIHI and Quebec are engaged in a process to make the data comparable and expect to have results soon (Leveille 2010, personal communication). Part of the explanation for Quebec's lower costs is that some medically necessary test are done in for-profit labs and not publicly reimbursed. Even if a reasonable estimate of such payments to private labs is included, and it is assumed that all tests are essential, it would still only bring Quebec's per capita cost up to $67. It seems likely that Quebec's low per capita cost is due in significant part to it being one of the more integrated and wholly public laboratory systems.

Head-to-Head System Comparisons

Even though direct comparison of the costs between hospitals and for-profit laboratories is not the real issue for the government in determining the most cost-effective method of delivering laboratory services, over the decades, many studies have used this approach. All of these analyses have been fraught with

Table 7-1   Government Per Capita Medical Laboratory Expenses by Province
(Actual dollars)

Province	1990/91	2001/2	2006/07
British Columbia	77	116.16	141
Alberta	91	74.40	123
Saskatchewan	74	73.62	118
Manitoba	75	77.97	110
Ontario	100	90.41	128
Average		77.49	108
Quebec	70		61
New Brunswick	51		105
Nova Scotia	74		105
Prince Edward Island	46		90
Newfoundland	NA		100

Sources: 1990/1 (Ontario Ministry of Health 1993e); 2001/2 (Bayne 2003); 2007/8 includes CIHI MIS data for hospital expenses. Added in BC were Medical Service Plan fee-for-service payments for diagnostic procedure codes 93 and 94; for Ontario added in are the public health laboratory expenses obtained from the Ontario Agency for Health Protection and Promotion and ohip payments for for-profit labs; in Manitoba the payments to the for-profit labs from Doctors Manitoba and the expense for the Cadham public health laboratory are included; Manitoba's figure is relatively low because the government was unable to provide the amount paid to small doctors laboratories or family physicians for providing laboratory services. For other provinces where doctors can bill health services for laboratory procedures it has been included in the per capita calculation. The Quebec figures are from Ministère de la Santé 2008.

difficulties because the two sectors provide different services, use different workload measurement systems and have different bottom lines. Nonetheless these analyses, which often show that public hospitals are no more expensive, give the most solace to the private sector.

Denis Fraser and Rick Lambert, in a 1991 paper prepared for the Ontario Society of Medical Technologists, compared the costs of laboratory tests from 1981/82 to 1988/89. Using raw data, total costs divided by the number of tests in each sector, they found that the average cost in the private sector was 33 percent higher than the average cost in a hospital.

The Ontario Ministry of Health has paid for four studies that tried to compare hospital costs with those of the commercial providers: a Woods-Gordon study of the HHSLP, the LOPPP review, a study conducted under the NDP's Social Contract legislation and a study by consultants Coopers and Lybrand in 1997. All are, to some extent, being kept secret.

I was unable to obtain a copy of the 1974 Woods-Gordon study, but it is described as an "inconclusive" study that tried to turn the hospital into a hypothetical private laboratory.[3] The LOPPP review was only made available after a Freedom of Information (FOI) request and even then substantial sections on cost were blacked out. The Social Contract study was never publicly released and no basic data related to it were found. Most, but not all, of the Coopers and Lybrand study was released to me after a two-year struggle with the Ministry under the FOI process.

The study undertaken as part of the NDP's Social Contract process and used by the supporters of the private labs as proof that they do it better highlights the problems with this approach. The final report was never publicly released yet it was widely available in policy circles. This study, like most others, starts with strong cautions about the results.

> The groups [in the external advisory committee] expressed concerns over the fact that various assumptions and generalizations had to be made, in the absence of accurate detailed data, in order to perform the analysis; and the possible biases thus introduced into the interpretation of results.
>
> Before commencing to discuss the results of the study, it is important to caution readers against simplistic interpretation of any of the analysis results, and to point out the need to recognize that there are methodological limitations preventing the generalization of some of the observations. (Ontario Ministry of Health 1994b: 2)

Virtually every figure in the report is shrouded in qualifications such as, "which may not be a true reflection of actual" and "these assumptions may not be valid in all cases." Dr. Mazzuchin, the technical director of Laurentian Hospital, called the report, "TOTALLY UNRELIABLE" (capitals in original).[4] No first level analyses or raw data were provided to support the findings. Comments from the OHA point out that the study rests on assumptions of a similar case mix between the community laboratories and the hospitals, which clearly doesn't apply, and attempts to derive real costs per unit rather than looking at the increased marginal costs of using the hospitals.[5] The Social Contract study, after decreasing the number of units counted in hospitals and increasing the overhead costs, found that the per unit costs in the hospital labs were higher than in the private laboratories. None of the problems with the report stopped the president of MDS (Chamberlain 1994) and government officials[6] from making general references to a study showing lower costs in the commercial labs to defend their 1996 moves to stop competition in the laboratory sector. This was similar to the use of the "mixed results" of the LOPPP evaluation in the 1980s to defend the expanded use of private corporations.

In 1997, the Ontario government commissioned Coopers and Lybrand (1997) to conduct a confidential review of the province's laboratory system. Part of the review found, after considering the problems of incomparable data and adding 25 percent to hospital costs for overhead and specimen procurement, that the cost per reported test in a hospital was $7.44 compared to $6.33 in a private laboratory. As well as numerous other problems, this study starts with the false assumption that hospitals and private labs have a similar test mix.

Head-to-Head Test Comparisons

Attempts have also been made to compare the costs of individual tests conducted in facilities with different ownership. In 1973, the Ontario government determined that the cost of providing serological tests for venereal disease in the public health laboratory was 50 percent less than using a private lab. Fraser and Lambert (1991) calculated the real cost of eight common laboratory tests done in a hospital and compared those findings to the LMS unit costs. They found that the cost per sample in a hospital was $3.14, compared to $6.22 in the private sector. The calculations for hospitals did not include any overhead costs. The Ministry of Health in Saskatchewan did a similar analysis on five common tests, but included overhead costs, and found that the provincial laboratory did the test for 25 percent of the fee-schedule rate charged by the private laboratories. More (1994) found that the cost of twelve common tests in Ontario's commercial sector was $128.22 compared to $76.93 in the Kingston General Hospital outreach program. An article in the *Globe and Mail* examining the rapidly rising costs of Vitamin D testing found that the private laboratories in British Columbia charged $94 per test, Ontario private labs $52, Ontario hospitals $32, and the Saskatchewan government lab did the test for $17 (Mittelstaedt 2010).

Why Are For-Profit Laboratories More Expensive?

There are a number of factors that explain why using for-profit corporations increases laboratory system costs. Some are specific to the way for-profits operate: an inflated fee-structure, delayed adoption of automation, fraud, profit-taking and conflict of interest. Other costs are incurred by the simple presence of a parallel for-profit sector providing the same service as public, non-profit providers. The lack of integration drives up system costs in a variety of ways, including excess capacity, extra governmental costs, excess administration and unnecessary testing. All these increase overall laboratory costs to the only payer, public insurance.

Inflated Fees

The unholy alliance between the medical profession and for-profit laboratories also manifests itself in an inflated fee structure. Historically, fee-for-service rates have been set by doctors' associations and bear little if any resemblance to the actual cost of conducting a test and maximum resemblance to the highest possible price that can be charged the public payer.

Concerns about the validity of Ontario's fee schedule have been widespread. As early as the 1970s, when a dispute between the federal government and Ontario led to an examination of fees for outpatient tests, it was found that the real cost in hospitals was 60.3 percent of the OMA fee schedule (Verbugge 1972). In 2005, Ontario's auditor general raised a similar concern that the province had not analyzed "the underlying actual costs of providing laboratory services" when they negotiated the fees paid to the private laboratories (Office of the Auditor 2005: 169).

Bayne (2003: 31) found a similar problem in British Columbia:

> The fee-setting process has not kept pace with developments in practice and changes in technology.... Fees that include an acquisition, technical and professional component are paid for many simple tests that are conducted on a single specimen and mechanically analyzed.... The current structure of setting outpatient prices [set exclusively by the affected specialty group, pathologists] contributes to growth in expenditures.

Fraud and Misuse

Billing for tests that were not done or unnecessary drives up costs. Some of the increased cost is the result of blatant fraud, for example, billing OHIP for tests that were not done (*Globe and Mail* 1977a). While this was rare, more common in the 1960's and 70s was the practice adopted by private labs of sending tests to a low-cost laboratory, usually the public health laboratory, and then billing medical insurance at the OMA rate (Chemical Engineering Research 1969).[7] Most of the extra cost from paying for tests that are not necessary is due to activities that, while not necessarily illegal, have only a "passing acquaintance" with the regulations.

As early as the 1960s in Ontario, excess usage was spurred by incentives from the for-profit industry that included cut-rate bargains, kickbacks, sweetheart rental arrangements and preferential service provision in exchange for more referrals. In one blatant example, a for-profit laboratory "offer[ed] bargain packages to physicians e.g., 25 tests for $50 or even $25, when 23 of the tests are neither indicated nor necessary."[8] In the last forty or so years, private companies in all provinces where they operate have been found, accused or rumoured to be providing inducements to physicians that add to the cost of laboratory services without adding to medical knowledge.

Profit

A common explanation of why commercial laboratory tests are more expensive is that they have to make a profit for their investors, and the three surviving corporations have been consistently profitable, regularly yielding over 8 percent per year on investments. A person close to the negotiations with British Columbia's for-profit labs in 2004 reports that the labs were forced to open their books, and the government calculated their profit rate at 44 percent. Ongoing profit rates are not easy to determine because the private ownership structure of most for-profit laboratories hides financial data, and data for the public corporations' Canadian operations is amalgamated into the overall company figures. But these are profitable companies and the profit is a real cost paid for by public dollars.

Excess Capacity

At the beginning of this chapter the argument was made that money could be saved by using the excess capacity in hospitals. Excess capacity is not just machinery and buildings. When there is a private laboratory operating parallel to a public hospital system, to say nothing of two or three competing private labs, each with its own CEO, human resource department and other administrative structures, all paid for by public health care dollars, costs go up (Fraser and Lambert 1991). One of the main reasons that U.S. health care is more expensive than Canadian is that, as a percentage of total costs, U.S. overhead expenses, mostly due to excess administration, are twice those in Canada (Angell 2008).

Excess Testing

To the cost of excess capacity and administration in systems using private laboratories is added the cost of excess testing resulting from a lack of integration. One cause of unnecessary testing is that tests ordered by family doctors and processed in laboratories outside of hospitals are then reordered by hospital staff doctors because they do not have access to the results of the first tests. If electronic health records ever become widespread, some of these problems will be reduced. But the introduction of electronic records in Ontario, as in other provinces, is being hampered by the number of providers that need to be integrated into one system. Most provinces already have, at least regionally within hospitals, a reasonable level of computerized laboratory information that is accessible to hospital staff. If hospital labs did all the community testing, as they do in the Atlantic Provinces, this kind of duplication would be significantly reduced.

Controlling excess utilization also means ensuring that only medically useful tests are ordered. As a starting point this requires that there is no incentive, either for the laboratory or the ordering physician, to increase quantity. Central to improving the appropriateness of tests is increasing contact between laboratory specialists and ordering physicians (Plebani 1999). Gamble (2002), in her study on public-private laboratory partnerships in Ontario, found that when the hospital lab work was moved off-site, laboratory specialists lost some of their influence over laboratory testing, which had a negative effect on quality. Programs to encourage appropriate ordering by family physicians in Ontario were only effective when the incentive for private laboratories to increase the number of tests was taken away. Also the fact that most private laboratories are not in the community where the tests are ordered exacerbates the problem of information flow between laboratory specialists, family physicians and patients, making it harder to ensure that only appropriate tests are ordered.

These problems are compounded by the conflict inherent in having laboratory specialists working in both systems. Specialists working in hospitals with connections to private laboratories have been accused of directing their hospital's work to their private laboratory, increasing the income of the private lab and increasing the cost to health insurance.

Further, unnecessary testing takes place when for-profit companies influence public opinion to pressure governments to pay for new screening programs or diagnostic tests that may not have been proven useful. Determining what test should be ordered and paid for out of the public purse is a complex political and technical discussion between the public and health care specialists. The presence of for-profit interests in the debate makes it more difficult to successfully resolve these issues in the public's interest.

Excess Bureaucracy

The use of for-profit providers results in unnecessary government bureaucracy. In Ontario, the Ministry of Health uses significant staff time to handle aspects of for-profit provision. The Ministry's staff negotiates agreements, sets fee schedules, monitors usage, reconciles payments, reviews licence applications and decides upon the location of specimen collection centres. None of this would be needed if all laboratory work was done in the public sector.

Two parallel systems can also be a problem in times of a health crisis. It is difficult enough to implement emergency plans within an integrated system with one administrative structure, but having to negotiate problems with multiple providers of essential medical services with different employers and bottom lines adds a potentially harmful level of complication. This was the situation in Ontario during the SARS outbreak when community collection centres were required for outpatient laboratory work, which meant making quick deals with the private laboratories. In the end the private laboratories said that the SARS crisis cost them over a million dollars and demanded a payment from the Ontario government of $350,000 for extraordinary costs (Ontario Association of Medical Laboratories 2003).

For-Profit Resistance to Integration

Numerous difficulties with coordinating, let alone integrating, the public and commercial laboratory systems have been identified: for example, the different purposes, methods of funding and of workload measurement, and the secrecy of the commercial sector. The evolution of these two systems in Ontario indicates that many of these differences served to isolate the hospitals and enable the commercial laboratories to freely expand and dominate the community market.

Further, there is an inherent bias in the private sector against integration. Integration is a winner-takes-all situation. In the end there will only be one provider, so all of the others lose whatever separate business identities they have developed. These concerns were expressed in the questions commercial companies raised in Ontario's 1999 RFP process. Sutherland (2007: 183) quotes a laboratory insider on the industry's view of integration:

> Needless to say the private sector did not like that process [the RFP]. There was lobbying to kill it.... you build up a business, you invest in infrastructure, in training staff, buying buildings and equipment... and someone who does not have any investments in the area if they are successful by undercutting you on an RFP, you have lost the entire investment in that area.... This is like a high-risk roll of the dice on

whether you are going to be in business or not [and] it is just far too
risky for anybody.

The Ontario for-profit laboratory industry welcomed being left out of the LHINs,
Ontario's regional health organizations, because they felt that the "economics
of the community sector requires provincial funding and provincial overview"
(Sutherland 2007: 183). The private laboratories in British Columbia and
Manitoba have also been able to escape integration into the regional health
authorities.

The for-profit laboratories' fears of integration may be justified. In 1995, the
Klein government in Alberta pushed most for-profit providers into consortiums
with the public sector to delivery regional services. All the involved companies
did lose their identities and, in exchange, gained greater access to impatient
laboratory work. Fifteen years later, most private sector labs have been closed
and most services have been brought back into the public sector.

What the Ontario experience indicates is that a commercial laboratory sector not only increases cost, but its existence blocks the integration of laboratory
services and whatever cost-savings that would bring about.

What Is the Extra Cost?

Some of the data on excess cost due to the use of for-profit providers comes
from times when payments to the industry were relatively unregulated. Since the
mid-1990s, all provinces that have private laboratories paid from government
funds have gained some level of cost control through cuts in fees and caps on
payments: changes brought about in large part due to the excesses under the
fee-for-service system. Ontario started with a cut of 11 percent in payments from
1992 to 1997, Alberta followed with a 45 percent cut in 1995, Manitoba with a
20 percent cut and British Columbia was the last with its 20 percent cut in the
fees paid to private laboratories in 2004. Saskatchewan brought most laboratory
services back into the public sector after 1995.

The long-term effect of these controls has yet to be determined. While the
rate of increase in payments to the private laboratory corporations has decreased,
costs related to excess capacity, excess administration, excess bureaucracy,
profit taking and unnecessary testing continue. It seems likely that the degree of
mitigation varies with the depth of integration and removal of the fee-for-service
incentive. These are moves that increase the likelihood, even from a straightforward management point of view, of the services simply being provided by the
public sector.

Many attempts have been made to arrive at the amount that system costs
have increased as a result of the use of for-profit laboratories. Not only is it
difficult to compare the costs in for-profit laboratories with the marginal costs
of increased hospital laboratory usage, but the other systemic costs associated
with for-profit use, excess administration, unnecessary government bureaucracy
and endemic over testing would be difficult to quantify without extraordinarily

detailed analysis of government and private corporation expenses. Regardless of the exact amount, it is clear that using commercial laboratories to provide publicly funded medical laboratory services is increasing health care costs. A practical example that gives an order of magnitude of the possible savings is the experience of the HICL in Ontario: using a non-profit community collection system and processing the samples in hospital laboratories cost about 75 percent of what was paid to the for-profit laboratories. Generalizing from this case, at least $250 million could be saved if all medical laboratory services in Canada were integrated into a public non-profit system.

Notes

1. "Memorandum re: Meeting with Executive of Ontario Medical Association – Wednesday, June 2/76 – 1530 Hours." AO, RG10 – 18, barcode 112932, box 2, file 0-128173.
2. "Hamilton Laboratory Funding Proposal," memo from P.J. Plant, Chief, Laboratory and Specimen Collection Center Inspection Service, to C.L. Brubacher, Director, Inspection Branch, April 5, 1978. AO, RG 10-39, file 57.01.01.
3. Ontario Council of Health, Meeting of the Task Force on Laboratory Services, Minutes November 30, 1981. AO, RG 10-247, container 1, Acc28303, B212530.
4. A. Mazzuchin, "Critique: 'Report of the Study on Costs and Implications of Transferring Laboratory Workload' (Social Contract Study, Laboratory Service Review)," December 12, 1995.
5. Ontario Hospital Association, "Response to Laboratory Services Review External Advisory Sub-Committee Social Contract Study Summary Report," Toronto, March 1994.
6. *Hansard*, 1996, Health Estimates Debate, February 15, Ontario legislature.
7. "Health Services Committee, 18 November 1974, meeting no. 2/74, minutes." AO.
8. "Common objective," memo from A.G. Gornall, Chair University of Toronto Department of Pathology, to D.J. Twiss, Commissioner of Hospitals, September 22, 1969. AO.

Chapter 8

Quality and Accessibility

While the focus of this book has been on ownership, cost and integration, quality and accessibility are also affected by funding and organizational structure. Although not meant to be a comprehensive review of the impact of ownership on quality or accessibility, the following comments highlight how quality and accessibility are related to ownership and funding.

Quality

Lillian Bayne (2003), in her review of British Columbia's laboratory system, identified three phases of laboratory services that require quality monitoring. First is the pre-analytic: Was the right test ordered? Was it needed? Was the sample properly identified, taken correctly and sent to the laboratory in a timely manner? Second is the analytic phase, the procedures in the laboratory: Did the analysis produce a correct result? Finally, there are post-analytic concerns: Was the result conveyed in a timely manner to the proper health care professional? Was it interpreted and used correctly? Mario Plebani (1999), taking a similarly systematic approach, identifies two important principles affecting medical laboratory quality. First, laboratory services need to be seen as a medical discipline whose clinical aspects are as important as, if not more important than, it's technical aspects. This means ensuring that the right test is ordered for the right patient and the results are used correctly. And second, the quality of medical laboratory services is dependent upon the interaction between medical laboratory specialists and health care providers outside the laboratory.

Quality Assurance Limited to Analytic Concerns

Most quality assurance programs in Canada focus only on the analytic, or technical, aspects of laboratory work: Did the analysis produce an accurate result? The key function of Ontario's external quality assessment program is "the assessment of laboratory test performance and education" (QMP–LS 2008). The introduction of an accreditation program in 2000 broadened the test of quality to include the management of the laboratory, but the focus is still on the running of the laboratory facility, particularly the testing procedures, and there is no consideration of systemic quality issues. Bayne (2003: 8) identified a similar limitation in British Columbia's quality assessment: "Only technical quality is formally measured… making it impossible to determine if patients are getting too many tests, the right tests, or tests at the right time."

One possible effect of limiting evaluation to the technical quality of laboratory testing is that official evaluations will likely find little difference between non-profit and for-profit labs. More (1994) makes the argument that technical quality is dependent upon the technology used, which is often similar in public and private sector laboratories. When other aspects of quality, for example, integration, access and appropriate testing, are excluded from the quality equation, the results of evaluation favour for-profit delivery. By removing from formal scrutiny the aspects of service provision that are affected by ownership, the impact of the use of private companies on quality is hidden.

Quality Assurance Limited by Secrecy

While More might be right that ownership has little effect on technical quality, in Canada there is no way to know for sure. In all provinces with for-profit laboratories, the outcomes of laboratory quality evaluations are shrouded in secrecy. Data that are made public are usually aggregated at a high level of abstraction, and more detailed results, if they are available at all, are usually only available for public sector labs.

That the existence of the private sector limits access to quality data was made apparent in a CBC exposé on the quality of laboratory services in Manitoba. A Freedom of Information request led to the release of documents revealing a series of quality problems in the public sector laboratories, but the investigators were not able to win the release of information on the quality of the private labs (CBC News 2008). Private labs in Manitoba are primarily paid by public dollars to deliver an essential medical service, but the public is not allowed to know whether they are producing quality results.

Ontario's Laboratory Proficiency Testing Program (LPTP), now the Quality Management Program–Laboratory Services (QMP–LS), argues that this confidentiality helps to ensure the cooperation of laboratory directors. This argument rests on the unsavoury assumption that even if it is a legal requirement, laboratory owners would not participate fully in a quality assessment if there is a chance that their lab, or even their sector, might be identified. Access to information on Ontario's quality program was further restricted in 2004 with the passage of the *Quality of Care Information Protection Act*. This act removed many aspects of the QMP–LS from the provincial auditor's oversight. In 2005, Ontario's auditor general lamented: "We were therefore unable to determine whether the quality-management program for laboratory services was functioning as intended" (Office of the Auditor 2005: 167).

The secrecy surrounding the quality of Ontario's laboratories contrasts with the Ontario Liberal government's program to publish hospitals' infection rates, mortality ratios and hand-washing compliance. In May 2010, Ontario's Liberal government announced it would be introducing the *Excellent Care for All Act,* which promises to open up public facilities to more scrutiny, which will widen the accountability gap between them and for-profit providers. The Act might more appropriately be called the *Excellent Care for all Except Those Who Use Private Facilities Act.*

Information on quality has not always been so secret. Ontario's early quality assessment programs produced yearly reports in which the results of assessments were presented by type of ownership and size of hospital. Between 1974 and 1984, the LPTP identified forty-two hospital laboratories, twenty-two private laboratories and two publicly owned laboratories as non-proficient. One private laboratory was closed as a result.[1] All the other laboratories were subjected to remedial action, such as discontinuing certain classes of tests, selling the laboratory or conversion of the lab to an SCC. Most of the hospitals that were found deficient were small and rural. This reveals little about the quality of the work of private compared to public operators; it only suggests that larger facilities are more reliable than smaller ones.

The problem of quality concerns in smaller hospital laboratories has been significantly eased by regionalization initiatives. A well-documented example is the Clinical Laboratories of Eastern Ontario, which was established as a network of nine hospitals, most small and rural, using the Kingston General Hospital (KGH) as a reference laboratory and quality centre. Laboratory specialists at KGH assist the smaller hospitals with quality programs and provide 24/7 consulting services on quality issues (More, Sengupta and Manley 2000). The program is now called the South-Eastern Laboratory Association.

The Medical Profession and Quality Monitoring

The secrecy around the quality of laboratory services is supported by the medical profession, which, in all provinces with a vibrant for-profit sector, polices laboratories. In the four western provinces, the College of Physicians and Surgeons runs the quality monitoring program. In Ontario, the control of doctors is even more direct. The profession's own association, the OMA, runs the program. The licensing and quality programs administered by the Ontario Medical Association tightly guard their data. Not only is this information not available to the public, even the Minister has for decades had difficulty getting access to it. In the mid-1980s the Ministry formally complained to the OMA that it was not receiving access to this information,[2] and the lack of accountability of the OMA to the government for laboratory quality was noted as a problem by Ontario's auditor general in 2005 (Office of the Auditor 2005). Nonetheless the government has not removed the OMA as the quality arbiter.

Even though most private laboratory services are now delivered by large corporate enterprises, there are still strong connections between these companies and the medical community. Historically, many laboratories were owned by physicians, and all labs still have to have medical directors who have a legal responsibility to maintain quality. This legal responsibility is tempered by the fundamental reality that the primary responsibility of for-profit corporations, which employ these doctors, is profit, regardless of who is managing quality. Senior managers in the Ministry of Health recognized this conflict as early as 1979:

> In cases where the owner and the pathologist (laboratory director) are different people… the pathologist must be prepared to place his professional reputation as well as his tenure of employment in jeopardy….

> Due to the corporate nature of ownership presently existing in the private sector, it is extremely difficult to place ultimate responsibility on the owner or to make the pathologist responsible in that he can always say he was carrying out the orders of the owners/owners. (Gold, Plant and MacKillop 1979: 6)

While it is likely that most doctors act in an ethical manner, clearly some do not, and the record of professional self-policing is, at best, clouded. A 2009 *Times-Colonist* article on quality in Canada's medical laboratories system notes that, "there is a long history in Canada of [medical] professional bodies hesitating when firm action was required." The medical community's tendency to secrecy reflects a bias towards private health care, and some doctors argue that their commitment to the Hippocratic oath removes the need for public scrutiny of their practices.

Quality in Ontario Labs

Despite the increasing secrecy there is some recent data available on the technical quality of Ontario's laboratories. Ontario's auditor general reported an error rate of just over 1 percent of all tests in 2004. "Significant errors," Ontario's quality management program's (QMP–LS) term for errors that could cause harm, rose by 23 percent from 2003 to 2004 (Office of the Auditor 2005). Considering the level of automation, the importance of test results and the testing conditions, these figures should be a source of concern. Errors were found, the auditor noted, in spite of the lenient conditions under which the evaluation was done: labs were given advance notice of the testing, and the samples were identified ahead of the test. After 2004, the QMP–LS's reports no longer provided detailed information on total errors or significant errors, so it not possible, even at this level of gross data, to evaluate changes in technical quality. The auditor also reported that some firms have continued processing tests with high error rates for decades and have not been shut down; nor is there a record of notification being given to patients who might have received faulty results. At last reporting, the Ontario government still has not moved to rectify these problems.

The increased secrecy and lack of accountability of our for-profit laboratories reflect the increased power of corporations in the neoliberal world. The role of capitalist governments to protect private interests, in this case through assuring business confidentiality, is strengthened as the power of private capital has made appeasing for-profit corporate interests more crucial.

Even though existing quality programs have significant problems arising from their secrecy, their limited focus and their conflict of interest from self-monitoring, their major harm may be that they deflect attention from systemic factors that affect quality, specifically problems arising from the lack of integration and lack of funding.

Pre- and Post-Analytic Quality — Resources and Integration

Across Canada the inability of laboratories to share data with other labs and with ordering physicians has been identified as a quality concern (Office of the Auditor 2005; Bayne 2003; Dalton 2010, personal communication). This issue has been raised in all provinces, so it is not entirely a problem of a having both public and for-profit laboratories working in the same market. Equally though, there seems little doubt that the existence of a private system does exacerbate the problem. The fragmentation due to parallel for-profit and non-profit laboratory systems and the private laboratories' role in maintaining that fragmentation is described in Chapter 4. The result is unnecessary testing, lack of timely reporting of test results, increased possibility of error in the transmission of results and an increase in the possibility that an important result will be missed.

In Ontario, the HICL pilot projects set up electronic access between the hospital laboratory and the area physicians; consequently, samples were quickly transported to a hospital lab and results were quickly available to the ordering physician (Silversides 2010, personal communication). This ended when the for-profits took over in these communities. Family doctors who had been used to receiving quick results from the local hospital laboratory now had to wait longer for results from the new for-profit provider. Ontario's HICL pilot projects produced results from the local hospital laboratory for most community patients within three to four hours compared to the twenty-four to forty-eight hours it takes the commercial labs (RPO Management Consultants 2008). A longer waiting time for a result negatively affects the quality of care patients receive. Also, because many kinds of samples deteriorate quickly or require storage at specific temperatures before analysis, the time required to transport samples to centralized facilities in another part of the province increases the possibility of an inaccurate result. As well, community doctors may now need to contact two providers, the hospital, if their patient has been an inpatient, and the for-profit lab, to obtain a full set of results for their patients.

When the pilot projects ended, patients also lost access to stat services. In Perth, Ontario, after Lifelabs took over community work from the HICL, patients who needed a stat INR, a blood test to determine how quickly bleeding stops, had their specimen sent to the Lifelabs facility in Belleville rather than the local hospital. "There is nothing stat about it," commented the Deborah Wilson, manager of a family health clinic (2010, personal communication). Now, if a patient needs a stat INR, Wilson's best advice is that the patient register as an outpatient in the Perth Hospital Emergency.

Brenda Gamble (2002) documented another problem associated with moving the site of processing away from the place of ordering, or as Plebani (1999) might say, when the interface between the immediate health providers and laboratory specialists becomes more difficult. In her case studies of public-private laboratory partnerships in Ontario, Gamble (2002: 108) found that clinical proficiency declined when the more automated services were moved away from the hospital:

> Due to the inability to fully interface the LIS [laboratory information
> system] with client hospitals and the location of the core laboratory off-
> site from the teaching hospital communication between the commercial
> laboratory and physicians and/or clients became lengthy and difficult.

A similar concern was raised by staff physicians in Edmonton's hospitals.
They reported difficulty accessing results and interpretations from an off-site
commercial lab, even with an integrated laboratory information system connecting the hospitals and the private lab. These concerns were part of the reason for
bringing the inpatient work back into the hospital and under hospital management in 2006 (Ballerman 2010, personal communication). In provinces where
hospitals process all the laboratory tests, while community doctors may not be
hooked into the hospital system, hospital staff doctors often have access to a
patient's full laboratory record, including tests ordered by the family doctor.
This reduces the number of tests and increases the accuracy of diagnoses.

Staffing is also a problem exacerbated by the existence of a parallel private
system. It is generally recognized that there is a shortage of skilled professionals,
from pathologists to laboratory technicians, throughout the laboratory system
(Carr 2003; Davis 2002). Multiple corporations and the public sector all competing for an already too small workforce decreases the efficient use of staff. As
well as not being able to adequately complete the work on hand, overworked
staff cannot keep up with the many new tests and technologies. To the extent that
having a stable, appropriately educated, motivated and well-resourced workforce
is important to quality this is a quality problem. The ongoing national discussion
about cancer pathology testing has identified the shortage of skilled pathologists and other laboratory professionals as one of the problems (Chorneyko
and Butany 2008; *CMAJ* 2008). Reports of quality problems in Manitoba's DSM
identify overwork as a key contributing factor, worsened by the fact that eight
of fifty-four pathology positions were vacant (Skerritt 2009).

Two broad themes that emerge from the steady stream of articles and letters in medical journals and newspapers on troubles in pathology in Canadian
hospitals are the lack of national standards and the under-resourcing of hospital
laboratories. Cutting the budgets of hospital laboratories as part of the neoliberal
restructuring of heath care services along business lines assumes that they are
"cost centres rather than patient-care centres" (Ford and Wadsworth 2008: 342).
This focus is particularly hard on resources for labour intensive tissue pathology
procedures, most of which are in the public sector and under pressure from the
"recommendations of consultants obsessed with centralization and automation"
(Ford and Wadsworth 2008: 342). The business model has also meant a decline
in the skill mix; laboratory technologists are being replaced with technicians
and technicians are being replaced with laboratory assistants.

There has always been a large discrepancy in staffing qualifications between
public and for-profit facilities. Public facilities hire proportionately more highly
trained technologists than technicians (Ontario Ministry of Health 1993b). This
is partially explained by the fact that hospitals do more technically demanding

work than the more standardized private laboratories, but it may also be because they operate under an ethos of service rather than an ethos of profit. To the extent that the decreasing qualifications of the workforce, in both for-profit or non-profit laboratories, is primarily budget related, it threatens quality.

The QMP–LS reports that most of Ontario's lab errors are caused by:

> [Lack of] accuracy and precision of automated systems and kit methods, and use of inadequate or outdated procedures or reporting protocols… failure to follow written procedures or survey instructions, incorrect instrument calibration, sample handling issues and failure to correctly interpret results. (QMP–LS 2008: 20)

It is easy to imagine that the qualifications of the staff, speed of work and profit motive are significant contributing factors to these problems. Wasting $250 million of our national laboratory spending on private profit and redundancies caused by the existence of for-profit services is a significant contributing factor to these quality problems. As Jason Ford and Louis Wadsworth (2008: 342) conclude, "this continual paring of laboratory budgets often leads directly to poorer quality care for Canadians, including misdiagnoses, miscommunications, medical errors, longer turnaround times for results and inappropriate therapies."

Access

The use of for-profit laboratories has had mixed effects on access. On the one hand, it has increased access for some patients. When fee-for-service payments were open-ended and there were limited controls on conflict of interest, access for many patients improved. In some communities there was a specimen collection centre in every doctor's building and on many neighbourhood corners, including locations that contravened government policy and compromised ethical and quality standards. When funding allowed the for-profits to maximize their income by maximizing the number of tests they processed, they made sure that everyone that could be profitably tested was. In some ways this is analogous to the situation in the United States. One of the reasons that Americans with money have good access to health care is that along with a chicken in every pot they have an MRI scanner in every neighbourhood. Unlimited access to funding breeds excess capacity and improved access for some patients.

Limited Access by Location

Even when for-profit services were expanding and funding was generous, for-profits limited access for some patients. In Canada, universal medical insurance removed the financial barrier to access… as long as you live in a high volume community. The neglect of rural regions by the for-profit sector was noted as early as 1973. In Toronto there were almost four and a half times as many commercial laboratories as hospital laboratories; in Northern Ontario there were three times more hospital laboratories than commercial laboratories. The pattern persisted into 1993, when Toronto had 83 for-profit laboratories, 158 SCCs and

Table 8-1   Geographic Distribution of Ontario's Medical Laboratories, 1973

Area	Hospital	Commercial	% Commercial
Metro Toronto	34	150	82
Central	44	60	58
Southwest	28	44	43
Southeast	36	29	45
Northern	42	13	24

Source: "Amendments to the Public Health Act relating to Laboratory Licensing: Summary," Cabinet Submission from the Ministry of Health, November 1, 1973, p. 5. AO, RG 10- 18, barcode 112932, Box 2.

58 hospitals, while Ontario's Northwest had 16 hospital labs, 4 public SCCs, only 5 for-profit labs and no private community SCCs (Ontario Ministry of Health 1993a). Similarly, the private laboratories in British Columbia shifted most of their work to the lower mainland, leaving the provision of service in the interior and the north mainly up to the hospital system.

The for-profit laboratories not only ignored the smaller communities but they actively undercut the public provision of services. The 1982 Task Force on Laboratory Services was

> concerned that referrals [by private laboratories] of routine testing out-side the county [rural areas] reduces the workload in small laboratories and increases it in large laboratories. It is detrimental to the maintenance of a sufficient volume of testing by the smaller laboratories to support appropriate laboratory manpower and methodology (e.g. automation). (Ontario Council of Health 1982: 144)

Removing services from smaller communities to feed the larger centralized private laboratories continued with the closure of Ontario's pilot projects and the downsizing of many smaller hospital laboratories, which negatively affects dozens communities. In Picton, for example, when the hospital laboratory was closed to community patients and replaced by Lifelabs, community access to an SCC fell from twelve hours a day to four. Community patients also lost their 24/7 access through the emergency department for more urgent tests (Renoy 2010, personal communication). For-profit companies are loath to bear the cost of providing access to rural populations. Maintaining a critical mass of staff and a reliable specimen transportation system in rural areas limits the potential for cost savings resulting from centralization (Bayne 2003). Manitoba has maintained rural access and maximized cost savings by only using the non-profit DSM to provide all laboratory services outside of Brandon and Winnipeg (Dalton 2010, personal communication). Access for patients in rural areas and smaller communities is a problem left to the public sector.

Limited Access to More Complicated Tests

For-profit laboratories will preferentially perform only the most profitable tests and leave the harder work to the public system: a practice known as high-grading or skimming. High-grading was already evident in 1969, when private laboratories performed 8 percent of all the laboratory work and 12 to 15 percent of the biochemistry, urinalysis and haematology, the simpler, more profitable tests (Chemical Engineering Research 1969). All major reviews of laboratory services in the western provinces and Ontario have found a similar phenomenon — the complicated, more labour intensive tests are left for the public sector to perform.

When for-profit labs pick and choose only the most profitable tests, access suffers. Patients may have to go to more than one site to have blood taken or wait longer for results. Instead of sending their samples to a hospital laboratory, which is likely closer, the sample might have to be sent to the central private laboratory, often in a different city, with longer turnaround times. This was my experience working on the VON's IV team. At the same time that the private corporations have been free to skim the easier tests, hospitals are expected to carry the brunt of the more complicated test with fewer resources. This is a characteristic of neoliberal restructuring of essential public services to boost private profit and undercut the ability of the public sector to deliver a quality service.

Limited Access for Marginalized Patients

In the face of funding restrictions, the for-profits cut back on access even in the more populated areas. Access has been reduced for all patients and people with mobility problems, and nursing homes have been the hardest hit.

In all provinces with for-profit services, the number of access points to laboratory services has decreased. The most dramatic reductions were in Calgary and Edmonton after the 1996 laboratory funding cuts. While access for community patients has decreased in Ontario, the pattern is different than in the western provinces. The number of SCCs connected to for-profit laboratories continued to increase as the number of laboratories decreased. But access to many of these centres has been limited, with reductions in SCC hours, reductions in staff and longer line-ups.

More important is that community patients in Ontario lost their access to hospitals for specimen collection. As a matter of right, before 2008 patients could go to their local hospital and have their blood taken. Since hospitals are widely distributed around the province, including in many smaller and northern communities, the ending of this practice has meant a reduction of 225 access points, and thus has limited access to all patients. Those communities with small populations have been hit the hardest.

Cross-province hearings held by the Ontario Health Coalition in 2010 documented these changes in many communities (Ontario Health Coalition 2010). For example, deputations at the Burkes Falls meeting reported that since the Huntsville Hospital was closed to community patients in 2008, there has been an increase in reports of late and inaccurate lab results:

On several occasions blood tests for Coumadin for one witness have gone missing and been as late as ten days. Previously, when lab work was done in Huntsville, his doctor got the results the same day.

Another witness described his experience with a rare myeloproliferative blood disorder of the bone marrow. If blood tests are delayed, he does not get accurate counts. He is on several medications. To overcome this problem, he would have his blood test taken in Burks Falls lab just prior to pick up time so that it was processed in Huntsville within a couple of hours. Since testing is no longer done in Huntsville, his blood is now sent to [a for-profit lab in] Brampton and there is a delay of up to 24 hours between the time blood is taken and testing is done. His blood tests are now inaccurate and have led to unnecessary changes in medication. (98)

Ability to Pay

Most laboratory services for tests that are listed as medically necessary are provided by our universal medical insurance system as a matter of right to all patients. Restrictions in funding to hospitals and permissive government attitudes have started to create differential access based on the ability to pay. New Brunswick and Nova Scotia, by not properly funding accessible community collection centres, have allowed unregulated for-profit companies to establish specimen collection services that provide better access to laboratory services for those who can pay. Reductions in the public sector have facilitated the expansion of for-profit services.

The existence of a parallel for-profit laboratory system also decreases pressure on the public system to provide tests since those with money can purchase tests that a doctor may consider necessary but that are not yet covered by public insurance. For instance, in Ontario, if a doctor thinks a patient needs a blood test for celiac disease, potentially gaining access to a diagnosis that can reduce years of suffering and the possibility of fatal cancers, patients with financial resources can pay a private laboratory $125 for the test, those with private insurance might be considered, and others have to go without because that cannot afford to pay. Restrictions on what is covered by the public system increase volume for private laboratories, increase the market for private insurance companies, limit the public system and harm those with fewer financial resources.

Conclusions

There is a tension between increasing accessibility, reducing cost and the ordering of unnecessary tests that needs further study. For instance, for-profit laboratories, to increase volume, increased specimen collection services. These services were rightly welcomed by patients but also increased cost and likely decreased quality through unnecessary testing. On the other hand, the private sector has shown a consistent reluctance to deliver equitable access to laboratory services to rural patients, marginalized patients and patients with complex needs.

The presence of for-profit laboratories has hurt quality by fragmenting the system and squandering resources. The monitoring of quality is suspect because of its lack of transparency and because of the self-serving relationship between the private labs and the medical profession. Systemic secrecy has decreased the accountability of for-profit laboratories.

For-profit provision of laboratory services raises legitimate concerns about quality and access. In spite of a common assumption that the private sector does things better, there is a lack of evidence that this is the case in laboratory services. Instead, there is growing evidence that corporate laboratories cost more than and do not serve patients as well as non-profit providers.

Notes

1. "*Globe and Mail* Request for Interview on Private Laboratories," Laboratory Services Branch, Ministry of Health, May 8, 1984. AO, RG 10-39, box 5, b383120.
2. "Assistant Deputy Minister's Briefing Book: Ontario Medical Association Laboratory Proficiency Testing Program (OMA-LPTP)," 1985. AO, RG-39, box 5, B383120.

Chapter 9

Physicians, Political Process and Private Profit

The For-Profit–Non-Profit Debate

When the *Medical Care Act* was enacted in 1968, all provinces had a comprehensive network of non-profit laboratories based in public hospitals and public health facilities. Five provinces allowed small for-profit laboratories to receive public money for providing essential laboratory services.

Forty-two years later, non-profit institutions are still the backbone of Canadian medical laboratory services. For-profit companies have expanded and consolidated; in 2010, they will be paid about $1 billion from public health care budgets. In Ontario, three multinational corporations dominate 50 percent of the laboratory market and supply most of the private medical laboratory services in Canada. Community laboratory systems range from exclusively public in the Atlantic Provinces to primarily for-profit in Ontario and British Columbia.

In spite of the provincial variation, this study highlights some common findings central to the larger public-private debate over the delivery of health services.

- For-profit laboratories capable of delivering a significant portion of essential services would not exist without substantial public support. They rely upon governments for funding and to create a market for their services, a policy that involves restricting non-profit public providers.
- The organized medical profession played a critical role in the development and defence of for-profit laboratories.
- For-profit laboratories work for their own profitability and work to undermine the public sector services in order to increase their market share and profit. Allowing for-profit provision made it more difficult to develop and implement policy in the public interest.
- The existence of for-profit laboratories increases the total cost of laboratory services and makes the integration of services more difficult.
- Allowing a parallel for-profit laboratory system hurts overall system efficiency.
- Improved access for all Canadians is not possible without public, non-profit health facilities and a universal health care system. For-profit companies only increase access to services where it is profitable.
- The technical quality of laboratory services is difficult to evaluate because of business confidentiality and because the medical profession shields for-

profit laboratories. The existence of a parallel private laboratory service has a negative effect on the quality of the laboratory system as a whole.

- Hospitals need on-site laboratories, and meeting the needs of acute care patients has not proven to be a profitable activity for private corporations.

These results of the forty-two-year experiment with publicly funded for-profit laboratory services provide a strong warning against permitting even small private companies to deliver essential health services.

Why Do We Have For-Profit Laboratories?

Faced with the many problems associated with using private corporations to deliver an essential medical service, problems that have been widely recognized across the country, and no significant benefits, many provincial governments still allowed and facilitated their use. Why?

Analysis of the development of for-profit laboratory services reveals a history that is non- linear and often paradoxical. All provinces have experienced pressure from the for-profit corporations for a slice of the province's laboratory money and increased pressure from the business community to control government spending. Federal government programs created and secured a strong public laboratory system and funded large for-profit laboratory corporations. And the medical profession played a major role in securing private, for-profit laboratories that ultimately undercut the power of doctors and diminished the value of the pathologist's work.

Two themes recur in this narrative that help to explain the success of for-profit laboratory corporations. First, mechanisms of the daily workings of government that tend to promote private profit over collective services played a central role. There is no level playing field. This bias is particularly apparent when there is no strong popular struggle to resist it: a force which, except in a few local instances, has been missing in the case of Canada's medical laboratory services. The effect of favouring the use of private laboratory corporations is that, as the use of private companies increases, the state's propensity to facilitate private profit over the public interest increases. Deciding to use for-profit corporations is not benign. These corporations become a force that decreases our governments' ability to make decisions in the public interest.

Second, aspects of biomedicine, the dominant ideology of medical practice in Canada, played a pivotal role in fostering the rise of for-profit laboratories. Doctors' professional organizations are the most visible manifestation of this phenomenon, but the standardized work and quantitative focus that is the bread and butter of the for-profit sector is strongly supported by allopathic practice.

Secrecy

Across the country, communities are having their laboratory services cut and restructured. When private companies deliver these services, we often have no control over what is cut, how much the administrators and staff of the corporations are paid, how much is transferred to shareholders and how much is used for new technologies. We do not know the terms of the agreements between these companies and governments, health authorities and hospitals. We often do not even know if contracts with private corporations exist or what services are involved. We do not know how safe these companies are, yet we are getting play-by-play updates on the safety of public hospitals.

The presence of commercial corporations in the laboratory sector created significant problems for data collection in Ontario. Without extensive access to information, the possibility of a full and informed debate on matters of public policy, a hallmark of any well-functioning democracy, does not exist. The problem is particularly troublesome when it affects our ability to participate in policy decisions central to the public's welfare, such as those affecting our health.

Ontario's Ministry of Health and Long Term Care, bolstered by section 17(1) of the *Freedom of Information and Privacy Act*, initially refused to reveal how much was paid by the medical insurance plan, OHIP, to the private laboratory corporations. The Ministry also denied access to recent studies on the laboratory industry, results on quality monitoring, information on how much was paid to the private sector lobby group for research and how it was spent, and details on specific contracts with private sector firms. Section 17(1) excludes from public discussion information that contains scientific, technical, commercial or labour-relations information provided in confidence to the government when disclosure of that information might harm the company.

Section 17(1) has also been used by the for-profits to restrict information on the location of laboratories and specimen collection centres, matters that by regulation are to be decided by the government based on public interest criteria. During the most recent provincial integration initiatives, one laboratory argued the following in a brief to the information and privacy commissioner: "A competitor, if aware that particular tests were not performed by [our lab], could take commercial advantage of this information by offering to provide a complete spectrum of all tests including those test [sic] that [our lab] does not perform, thereby resulting in direct loss to [our lab's] revenues" (Information and Privacy Commissioner 2003). For-profit laboratories were also reluctant to provide information to assist with Ontario's various regionalization processes. If for-profit companies are not willing to even reveal what tests they perform, then the prospects for integration of the services provided by these organizations are very dim.

The Freedom of Information process also strongly favours private companies. As a lone, unpaid researcher with a limited legal background, I entered the appeal ring against a bank of law firms paid by the for-profit companies, to say nothing of the thousands of public dollars spent by the Ministry to resist giving access to information.

Some hospitals have been equally reluctant to provide details about partnerships and contracts they have with for-profit firms (Gamble 2002). And the companies themselves have no obligation to provide data except as required by security regulators. This means there is very little public information about any of the laboratory companies in Canada. Most are subsidiaries of larger companies, and details about provincial or Canadian operations are subsumed in general company information, or they are private corporations that are required to make very little data public. A level playing field between for-profit and non-profit providers is not possible because of the secrecy that surrounds the operations of the publicly financed for-profit providers.

Unequal Standards of Proof

In Ontario, private laboratories were allowed to develop in part because it could not be proved unequivocally that the public sector provides a superior service. As the decades passed, more and more effort went into manipulating studies to show that using hospital laboratories might not save money. Not only did the private sector stretch the truth to their benefit when interpreting studies — for example, in their use of both the Social Contract study and the LOPPP evaluation — but they intervened to stop evaluations that looked likely to produce evidence contrary to their interests. The LOPPP study was ended early, and in 1977 the OAML talked the Ministry out of studying the cost of providing the twenty most common tests in hospitals versus private labs.[1] This lack of hard data was then used to defend the practice of using private laboratories to deliver publicly funded services. The opposite, though, is not true. Having strong evidence and arguments in favour of using the public sector for all laboratory services does not guarantee that governments will take that route.

This unequal burden of proof is premised on the belief that the private sector does it better, a bias central to the functioning of market-driven societies even when there is no evidence to support it. The underlying bias is not only strong enough to often motivate governments to choose these companies over non-profits in a situation where it is a toss-up between the two, it has also overcome significant evidence that using for-profit providers is a bad idea.

Unequal Voices

For-profit corporations are permitted to publicly influence the political process through political donations and lobbying in a manner that is not allowed to the public sector. The links between for-profit corporations and government bodies that affect laboratory policy, whether it is managing hospital laboratories, provincial laboratory systems or regional health authorities, are legion in the history of medical laboratory services. These kinds of conflicts of interest that allow laboratory specialists to participate in public policy decisions affecting companies they are connected with is partially a residual benefit of the belief that doctors will act only in the interests of their patients. It is assumed that doctors are above the temptation to work for their own private profit. The private laboratories enjoy both the power of public lobbying and that of being able to make economic threats that are not easily available to the public and non-profit providers.

Private Profit versus Public Interest

As for-profit laboratories grew, they became more deeply integrated as stake-holders into the government decision-making processes. Yet their bottom line depends on running a profitable company, not working in the public interest. In the end, if they do not protect their private interests, they cease to exist.

For-profit companies actively lobbied against hospital laboratories doing work that they could profit from, undermined integration efforts and used their influence to end viable non-profit laboratories. In Ontario, a separate workload measurement and funding system was developed for the for-profit laboratories that increased their income, discouraged automation and further separated them from the hospital sector.

The confounding and perverse influence of private interests and the fee-for-service system on valuable social goals can be seen in the licensing and conflict-of-interest initiatives in Ontario. Increasing access, increasing test accuracy, integrating laboratory records and limiting fraud and unnecessary testing are generally accepted as positive social goals. Yet policies designed to realize these goals can be called into question when private providers stand to lose from the way the policies are implemented. Are the polices being skewed to increase private profit? Would the policies be stronger and more effective if we were only concerned about the public interest rather than insuring that a private company can also make a profit? The presence of a profit motive makes it difficult to gain the benefit intended by public interest policies. These concerns do not arise when there are no for-profit corporations competing with public sector providers.

Corporations are free to invest the profits made from our public payments as they wish. These companies use income from public sources to push for more private health care, both through direct lobbying and through the funding of companies that make pharmaceuticals and medical equipment and provide private diagnostic services and for-profit home care. In essence the government has given private investors large sums of public money to invest as they see fit, creating a situation in which there is a serious lack of accountability in the use of public funds.

The Medical Profession and For-Profit Laboratories

The rise of for-profit laboratories, and even their existence, was greatly aided by the actions of the doctors' professional associations, the Canadian Medical Association (CMA) and its provincial counterparts, the Ontario Medical Association (OMA), Doctors Manitoba, etc. The organizational power and authority of the medical profession kept laboratory services from being fully covered by universal hospital insurance. Doctors negotiated a separate market for community laboratory services and direct access to insurance funding for private laboratories. The medical profession worked hard to limit programs intended to improve quality, end conflict of interest and reduce utilization. But it is simply not enough to blame the rise of for-profit corporations on greedy doctors. While they do exist, the root of the problem is the core principles of the dominant approach to health care in Canada, biomedicine. The biomedical approach has both favoured the centrality of laboratory services and provided opportunities for private companies to deliver these services.

Biomedicine makes a privileged place for laboratory services. The allopathic approach identifies the cause of illness as an outside invader or an internal malfunction, both of which can be identified and then fixed by increasingly elaborate technological and systematic interventions. This favours the quantitative, scientific and technical approach of laboratory testing. This is the core of laboratory work. Labs reduce health problems to cells and numbers.

The routine nature of much laboratory work favours standardization of large volumes of many common tests: a key condition for the commodification of any service. The laboratory process lends itself to centralization. The equipment required to take most samples is simple, and samples can easily be transported to be processed away from collection sites. Processing can be centralized and specimen collection dispersed. This organization was further encouraged by automation, which, in order to be cost effective, requires large volumes of samples, and the development of better road and air transportation. All of these factors played a part in the evolution of large laboratory corporations.

Central to the beliefs of biomedicine is that doctors are the lynch pin of medical practice (Armstrong and Armstrong 2003). They are assumed to be the ultimate authority: not only do doctors know best but they only act in the interests of their patients. Many small, essentially unregulated laboratory companies flourished under these conditions and, with expanding incomes from ever-larger insurance plans paying fee-for-service, grew into larger commercial operations.

Another component identified by Leys (2001) as necessary for the commodification of services is that "people must be induced to want to buy them." Doctors, who under biomedical norms are given the power to determine medical needs, are also often in a position to benefit from the expansion of these needs. Providing more medical technologies, including laboratory services, becomes a profitable dynamic reinforced by a model of health and treatment that focuses on the individual and technological interventions. Laboratory medicine is increasingly at the centre of this process. The recent push from private labs to increase DNA analysis, vitamin D level testing, measurement of the effectiveness of aspirin and population screening programs, all of which rely on laboratory services, exemplify this process.

While it is important to understand the aspects of biomedicine that favour turning an essential service into a commodity, this is not an attack on all the science, drugs and interventions developed under the biomedical model. Many medical advances, some obvious such as insulin, antibiotics and laboratory tests for a wide variety of disease-causing factors, have improved health. Laboratories played a key role in the early public health movements that lead to major increases in general population health. Regardless, uncritical acceptance of the biomedical approach and physician authority has worked fairly consistently against public health care services that meet population health needs and in favour of private, for-profit solutions.

Some Restrictions of For-Profit Delivery

It is important to note the reduction in the use of for-profit companies after the mid-1990s and its place in the history of their rise. Undoubtedly, for-profit corporations are still a significant factor in the delivery of laboratory services in Canada, but, even in Ontario, where they succeeded in ending non-profit community services, many of their links to inpatient services have been severed. Campaigns against the use of private laboratories led to the ending of private processing in Saskatchewan, and organized opposition in Ontario managed to salvage the non-profit pilot projects for a decade. For-profit advances to the Atlantic Provinces were rebuffed with resistance from both professional and community groups.

A significant source of opposition to the corporate laboratories came from within the medical community. Across the country, physicians, largely based in hospitals and worried about the threats to their autonomy and to the quality of service, publicly advocated for more resources for hospitals and greater restrictions on private laboratories. This opposition grew louder as the impact of for-profit laboratories grew. However, only rarely did the opposition call for an end to private provision. Rather, it argued for a level playing field between hospitals and private companies competing for community laboratory services — a playing field that cannot exist in a market-driven society. This physician opposition has had a limited effect in the provinces where for-profit delivery exists.

The major reason for the retrenchment of private laboratory services rests in a paradox of the neoliberal state. The excesses of the laboratory corporations, as they became more dominant in the provision of services, created financial problems for governments committed to shrinking the state, running the health care system as a business and reducing taxes. The excesses of one sector deriving its income from the public purse were becoming too much for the general interests of corporate Canada.

All provinces have introduced some form of regionalization as part of the restructuring of health services along business lines. For-profit provision has been most seriously curtailed in those provinces where laboratory services were regionalized and removed from provincial medical services. This is most notable in Saskatchewan and Alberta. Probably fearing the same result, the medical community and the private laboratories have fought inclusion in the regional health authorities in British Columbia, Manitoba and Ontario.

The jury is still out on the long-term effect of regionalization on for-profit laboratory services. The creation of integrated data networks and stand-alone laboratory corporations, which are the goals of many integration initiatives, could facilitate future privatization of some or all of these services. It could also form the basis of a more accessible and cost-effective public system. As with all reforms, they are multifaceted, and their effect is dependent on the strength of the various forces in our political economy.

How to Improve Laboratory Services

The first step in improving services is to do no more harm. As a matter of public policy, no increase in the amount and range of for-profit provision of laboratory services should be allowed, and where it can be done easily, services should be returned to the public sphere. After stopping the harm, one approach to improving service would be to integrate all laboratory services in a geographical area in a non-profit structure. Many services in most provinces currently approximate this approach. All medical laboratory services in rural and small communities in all provinces except Ontario are primarily delivered through the public system. In Quebec and the Atlantic provinces, all publicly financed laboratory services are non-profit. Ending fee-for-service payment and giving responsibility for delivering all laboratory services to one of the already existing regional or provincial authorities would make for a straightforward transition to a more integrated non-profit system in British Columbia, Alberta, Saskatchewan and Manitoba.

In Alberta all lab services are already coordinated under the Alberta Health Services Board. DynaLIFE, the only significant for-profit laboratory company in the province, provides services to the Edmonton area on a fixed-term contract. At the end of the contract, in 2016, these services could be moved back into the public non-profit sector relatively easily. If necessary some of DynaLIFE's facilities could be bought as was done when Calgary Laboratory Services purchased MDS's Calgary operations.

British Columbia has strong regional health authorities, which, if given appropriate increases in their global budgets, could provide all the laboratory services in their areas. Many hospitals already have processes in place for handling community work. Diagnostic Services of Manitoba (DSM) already delivers around 80 percent of that province's medical laboratory services. Either making DSM responsible for providing the remaining community work or shifting the responsibility for all laboratory services in Winnipeg and Brandon to their well-established regional health authorities, with corresponding funding increases, are viable alternatives. Saskatchewan could end the use of for-profit laboratory corporations by mandating that all the health authorities take over specimen collection.

Ontario poses the biggest political challenge. It is the heart of the beast: home of the largest for-profit laboratory corporations in Canada and the highest rate of private provision. It has the greatest for-profit influence on inpatient laboratory services, the medical profession and the Ministry of Health. On the other hand, it also has strong organized community voices that would support a move to provide all laboratory services through the public system and successful examples of how these services could be integrated into one system, i.e., Hamilton and the HICL.

As in British Columbia and Manitoba, an important first step in Ontario would be to end the fee-for-service system of payment for laboratory services and the provincial agreements with for-profit laboratories for delivering community laboratory services. All of the companies are covered under a negotiated contract with the Ministry of Health: at the end of the contract, the services could be moved back into the non-profit sector.

The first technical problem is the relatively new regional health organizations, the local health integration networks, the LHINs. The LHINs have been plagued with problems. Their size has been questioned, the Ministry has over-ridden their authority, they lack effective community control, their emphasis on centralization over service has been challenged and important aspects of health care, including community laboratory services, are not under their jurisdiction. Given the weakness of the LHINs, it might make sense to bypass them and re-invigorate the HICL community network, or set up another non-profit or public sector structure to do similar work. It would also be reasonable, and within the Ontario tradition, for hospitals to make proposals to collect and process community work in their regions. Hospitals and integrated hospital networks that are willing to take on community work could be identified. Extra funds could be funnelled to these facilities. As it becomes clear how much community work hospitals can take on, private sector facilities, if needed, could be purchased as contracts expire and integrated into the public system.

Also, with an infusion of relatively small amounts of money, it is likely that many communities would not only be able to move most community work into public sector laboratories but also provide community health care providers with direct links to the laboratory data. The 1998 pilot projects in Ontario were able to do this in the smaller communities they served. In Kingston, community health providers are already able to access the regional teaching hospital's medical records, including laboratory results. It would simply be a matter of extending this existing program. While OLIS, the province-wide laboratory information system, may have a few long-term advantages, most patients do not move from region to region and there are many easy successes to be had in regional information systems.

In Ontario's 1992 Laboratory Services Review, the expense of compensating the private laboratories for loss of business was raised as a reason to stay with the for-profit providers. This is a likely a red herring. This issue was dealt with in a 1998 court case against the Ontario government's regulation 02/98, which limited competition in the laboratory sector. The court ruled: "the Ministry was simply seeking an alternative to the fee-for-service system [and] there is little to support this claim to a vested right in a previous method of distribution" (Simpson 1999). For-profit laboratories are on time-limited contracts with no guaranteed volume of work. Buying out the businesses would probably not be necessary, although purchasing some facilities and equipment might make sense.

Many of the workers in the for-profit laboratories could find employment in the public sector and, unlike with most restructuring, the change in employment conditions in this case would be for the better. Whatever short-term transitional costs there might be would be recovered very quickly by the savings from a more integrated system.

The Problem of Specimen Collection

Moving to an integrated public sector system for laboratory services raises the issue of good access to specimen collection. Canada's existing non-profit laboratories, the ones that will be at the core of any integrated laboratory service, are based in institutions that are used to having patients come to them. The private laboratories have identified specimen collection as one of their strengths, and certainly the emergence of private phlebotomy services in the Atlantic Provinces and the continued use of a private provider in Regina and Saskatoon indicate a reticence on the part of some institutions to go out into the community to increase access.

On the other hand, the HICL, the Hamilton Health Sciences Laboratory Program, the Calgary Laboratory Services and many hospitals in British Columbia have demonstrated that hospital laboratories can be integrated with a system of community collection centres. It is really a matter of appropriate policy and funding of either hospitals or community oriented non-profit services like the HICL to provide these services.

Actions Speak Louder than Administrative Changes

The above administrative changes could help facilitate the development of a stronger public medical laboratory system able to meet a community's health needs. But, by themselves, they are limited and might facilitate the further privatization of health services. The structural changes need to be accompanied by political will and public pressure for no-profit service provision. Broader public debate on the problems of for-profit delivery of health care and on how to improve public services, including how to make them more open and democratic and less institutional, needs to take place. It must be recognized that all integration is not good integration. It needs to be implemented so that it increases access, quality, democracy and efficiency. Broad-based community organizations, such as the health coalitions and the Friends of Medicare, need to be supported and they need to organize communities to work for the public delivery as well as the public funding of all health services. The history of laboratory services argues strongly that the long-term ability to provide universally funded health care services relies upon them being publicly delivered.

Conclusion

The influence of a global economy in which capital mobility was increasing, from 1968 to the present, can be seen in changes in the provision of Canada's laboratory services. Governments shifted from supporting non-profit medical laboratory services to supporting more for-profit alternatives and the restructuring of non-profit services along business lines. Government secrecy increased. The power of the medical profession waned, with restrictions on fee-for-service payment and an increase in direct government and corporate control of service

delivery. There has been a loss of local service delivery and more centralization, often accompanied by a loss of access. While not always supporting the
direct access of private business to public money, the broader economic shifts
over the last four decades have seen a restructuring of health care services that
encourages more private accumulation of resources in the laboratory corporations and in the broader corporate community. This is the result of Ontario's
agreements with the OAML. These approaches have almost always resulted in a
reduction in service delivery.

While I was working on this book I received a call from a friend who still
works as a community care nurse. She told me about a series of cuts including
cuts to home care laboratory services. Her patients, many of them sicker than the
patients we were seeing fifteen years ago, who have chronic conditions requiring
frequent blood work, now have to go to a community specimen collection centre
or pay the private company a fee for at-home service. Also, with the closure
of hospitals to community patients, any of her patients requiring quick access
to blood results now have to go to a hospital emergency room and become an
inpatient. The access we had as home care nurses to hospital laboratories is now
gone.

Our local experience with home care laboratory services reflects the general
findings of this forty-year case study of for-profit delivery of medical laboratory
services in Canada. The practice of using for-profit laboratory corporations is
not acceptable in the provision of an essential service. Ownership matters. For-
profit provision costs more, negatively affects the pubic delivery of health care,
decreases quality, provides unequal access and limits democracy. Allowing for-
profit companies to provide a publicly funded essential service limits our ability
to build on our already strong non-profit laboratories to create the laboratory
system that is our best option for the future.

Note

1. M. Fournier, "Laboratory Co-ordination Activities as of June, 1978," memo to Dr.
    Aldis, June 26, 1978: 4. AO.

Personal Communications

Ballerman, Elisabeth, President, Health Sciences Association of Alberta.

Bonin, Raymond, retired pathologist, Laurentian Hospital, Sudbury, Ontario.

Buott, Kyle, Nova Scotia's Citizens Health Care Network.

Clarke, Lori, Laboratory Consultant, New Brunswick Department of Health.

Collins, Marilyn, Program Manager, Newfoundland and Labrador Provincial Blood Coordinating Program.

Connors, Kathleen, Chair, Canadian Health Coalition.

Crocker, Brian, Manager of Pathology Informatics, Capital District Health Authority, Nova Scotia.

Dalton, Jim, CEO, Diagnostic Services of Manitoba.

Harvey, Régis, Directeur Général, CSSS de Jonquière, Quebec (General Director of the Centre of Health and Social Services of Jonquière).

Hofer, Tammy, Acting Vice President, Laboratory Services, Alberta Health Services.

Jamieson, Roger, Compensation Analyst, Doctors Manitoba.

Jenson, Rick, Ontario Public Sector Employees Union.

Leveille, Pierre, Program Consultant, MIS & Costing, Canadian Institute for Health Information.

Levert, Elyse, Direction Générale des Services de Santé et de Médecine Universitaire, Province de Quebec.

Mallam, Katie, Communications Advisor, Doctors Nova Scotia.

Mason, Lori, Laboratory Manager, Laboratory Medicine Program, University Hospital Network, Toronto.

More, David, Manager, Kingston General Hospital Laboratory Services.

O'Brien, Fran, Administrative Director, Laboratory Services, Capital District Health Authority, Nova Scotia.

Ohmert, Ron, retired Research Director, Health Sciences Association of BC.

Perrins, Dan, Senior Fellow with the Johnson-Shoyama Graduate School and senior official in the Saskatchewan Minister of Health in the 1990s.

Prémont, Marie-Claude, Professeure Titulaire, École Nationale d'Administration Publique, Montreal.

Renoy, Pat, Picton Health Coalition and retired Registered Nurse.

Schatz, Diana, a microbiologist and Chair of Ontario's 1994 Laboratory Services Review.

Schneider, Dave, Laboratory Manager Queen Elizabeth Hospital, Prince Edward Island.

Silversides, Ann, freelance health journalist.

Simard, Louise, NDP Minister of Health in Saskatchewan, 1991–1995.

Smillie, Beth, Communications Representative, Canadian Union of Public Employees.

Steeves, Daryl, Administrative Director Laboratory Services, Horizon Heath Region, New Brunswick.

Swaine, Fred, CEO of the Eastern Ontario Regional Laboratory Association, Past COO, Calgary Laboratory Services.

Tajaja, Andrea, Coordinator Community Laboratory Services, Hamilton Regional Laboratory Medicine Program.

Tse, Leo, Manager, Licensing and X-ray Inspection, Ontario Ministry of Health.

Wilson, Deborah, Office Manager, Isabella Medical Clinic, Perth Ontario.

References

Angell Marcia. 2008. "Privatizing Health Care Is Not the Answer: Lessons from the United States." *CMAJ* 79, 9.

Armstrong, Pat, and Hugh Armstrong. 2003. *Wasting Away: The Undermining of Canadian Health Care*. Second edition. Toronto: Oxford University Press.

Austen, Ian. 1997. "Medicare? Gotta Love it." *Canadian Business* June.

Bator, P.A., and A.J. Rhodes. 1990. *Within the Reach of Everyone: A History of the University of Toronto School of Hygiene and the Connaught Laboratories*. Ottawa: Canadian Public Health Association.

Bayne, Lillian. 2003. *BC Laboratory Services Review*. BC Ministry of Health.

Bell, R. Edward. 1970. "Medical Laboratory Accreditation and Quality Control in Alberta." *CMAJ* 130 (November).

Berger, Darlene. 1999. "A Brief History of Medical Diagnosis and the Birth of the Clinical Laboratory: Part 4 — Fraud and Abuse, Managed Care and Lab Consolidation." *Medical Laboratory Observer* December.

Boyd, E.A.D. 1969. "Laboratory Utilization Study." OMSIP. Archives of Ontario.

Brain, M.C., R.A. Hagger, S. Moore, and R.W. Cameron. 1976. "The Hamilton District Program in Laboratory Medicine: A Progress Report on Integration." *CMAJ* 144 (April).

Brenblum, Edward G. 1998. "The Central Laboratory: Who Needs It?" *Medical Laboratory Observer* 30, 7 (July).

British Columbia Ministry of Health. 1993. *Review of Diagnostic Services: A Report to the Minister of Health Province of British Columbia*.

British Columbia Ministry of Health Services. 2010. *MSP Information Resource Manual: Fee-For-Service Payment Statistics — 2008/9*.

Bunting Peter, and Carl van Walraven. 2003. "Effect of Controlled Feedback Intervention on Laboratory Test Ordering by Community Physicians." *Clinical Chemistry* 50 (December).

Canadian Press. 2005. "MDS Inc. Agrees to Lab Unit Refunds: Americans Billed for Insured Tests: Up to 2 Million Claims Possible." June 30.

Carr, Nancy. 2003. "Dr. Dexter's Corner: Canada Faces Pathologist Shortage." *Pathology News* Queens University, Department of Pathology, March.

CBC News. 2008. "Problems Plague Manitoba's Medical Laboratories: Inspections Reports for Private Labs Not Available to Public." <cbc.ca/Canada/Manitoba/story/2008/02/06/lab-testing>. February 6.

CBC Web News. 2009. "N.L. Backs Down on Flower's Cove Cuts." October 23. <cbc.ca/canada/newfoundland-labrador/story/2009/10/22/nl-lab-xray-221009>.

Chamberlain, Art. 1994. "Provincial Report Backs Private Labs: Industry Relieved, Health-Care Unions Furious." *Toronto Star* March 28.

Chemical Engineering Research Consultants Limited. 1969. *Private Clinical Laboratories in Ontario: A Study for the Committee on the Healing Arts*. Toronto: Queen's Printer.

Chernos, Saul. 2009. "Speedy Lab Results: From Lab to Computer: Test Results are Flowing Electronically and Automatically." *Technology for Doctors* 5, 4 (October).

Chorneyko, Kathy, and Jagdish Butany. 2008. "Editorial: Canada's Pathology." *CMAJ* 178, 12 (June).

CLS and GSA Consulting, A Consortium of Laboratory Planning Specialists. 1994. "A Conceptual Framework for a Province-Wide Laboratory Services Delivery System." Laboratory Services Review, Ontario Ministry of Health.

CMAJ. 1971. "B.C.M.A. Advises Members of Stand Against Laboratory License Laws." *CMAJ* 105, 36 (August).

_____. 2008. "Canada Lags in Standardized Protocols for Medical Labs." *CMAJ* 179, 2 (July).

CML. 2001. *CML, Canadian Medical Laboratories: 2001 Annual Report: Strengthening Healthcare Services.*

CML Healthcare. 2009. *The Image Is Clear: CML Healthcare, Annual Report, 2009.*

CML HealthCare Inc. 2003. "CML Healthcare Announces 2003 Fiscal Year End Results and Proposal to Convert to an Income Trust to Enhance Shareholder Value." Media Release. December 16.

Cohen, Lynne. 1996. "Issue of Fraud Raised as MD Self-Referral Comes under Spotlight in Ontario." *CMAJ* 154.

Cole, James. 2004. "AIC Canadian Focused Corporate Class: A Management Discussion of Fund Performance." <aic.com/Resources/pdfs/en/can_foc_corp_ann_ENG_2004>.

Commission on the Future of Health Care in Canada. 2002. "Commission on the Future of Health Care in Canada: Open Public Hearing, Summary Notes: Regina, Saskatchewan — March 4, 2002." <http://www.collectionscanada.gc.ca/we-barchives/20071223015148/http://www.hc-sc.gc.ca/english/pdf/romanow/pdfs/regina_day_1_notes.pdf>.

Coopers and Lybrand. 1997. "Ontario Ministry of Health Laboratory Services Funding Models." Ontario Ministry of Health.

Corpus Sanchez. 2007. *Changing Nova Scotia's Healthcare System: Creating Sustainability Through Transformation: System-Level Findings and Overall Directions for Change, the Final Report: Provincial Health Services Operational Review (Phsor).* Nova Scotia: Department of Health.

_____. 2008. *An Integrated Health System Review in PEI: A Call to Action: A Plan for Change.* PEI Department of Health.

Davis, Kurt. 2002. "Responding to the Medical Laboratory Staffing Shortage: The Canadian Perspective." *Clinical Leadership and Management Review* 16, 6 (November/December).

Deber, Raisa. 2004. "Delivering Health Care: Public, Not-for-Profit, or Private?" In Gregory Marchildon, Tom McIntosh and Pierre-Gerlier Forest (eds.), *Romanow Papers, Volume 1: The Fiscal Sustainability of Health Care in Canada.* Toronto: University of Toronto Press.

Derfel, Aaron. 2005a. "Montreal Leads the Country in Offering Private Health Care: Parallel Medical Services a Way to Avoid Long, Sometimes Dangerous Waits." *Montreal Gazette* February 12.

_____. 2005b. "Doctors Probed for Kickbacks." *Montreal Gazette [Final Edition]* May 7.

Diekmeyer, Peter. 2003. "LDS Tests Positive for Success: Diagnostic Services Clinic Scores Big by Taking Hospital Overflow." <http://www.peterdiekmeyer.com/030915.htmlpeterdiekmeyer.com/030915>.

Donovan, Kevin. 1998. "Medical Labs Argue Against Payment Limits." *Toronto Star* November 26.

Erwin, Steve. 2004. "MDS Takes Big Writedown: Tide of Red Ink at Lab-Services Firm

Hits $36 Million Takes $63 Million Goodwill Charge on Stake in Subsidiary."
Toronto Star June 3.

Evans, Robert. 1993. "Health Care Reform: 'The Issue From Hell'." *Policy Options*
July August.

_____. 1997. "Going for the Gold: the Redistributive Agenda Behind Market Based
Health Care Reform." *Journal of Health Politics, Policy and Law* 22: 2 (April).

Fagg, Kelly L., Phil Gordon, Bonnie Reib, Joseph T. McGann, Thomas E. Higa, David
W. Kinniburgh, and George S. Cembrowski. 1999. "Laboratory Restructuring in
Metropolitan Edmonton: A Model for Laboratory Reorganization in Canada."
Clinica Chimica Acta 290.

Forbes, Jonathan. 1996. "Test Case: Private vs. Public Laboratories," Toronto: Ontario
Public Service Employees Union.

Ford, Jason, and Louis Wadsworth. 2008."Pathology Practice in Canada." CMAJ 179, 4
(August).

Fraser, Denis, and Rick Lambert. 1991. "Laboratory Out-Patient Funding: Past, Present
and Future." A paper presented to the Ontario Society of Medical Technologists'
28th Annual Convention, September 26.

Freedman, Theodore. 1970. "A Review of the Experience of the In-Common Laboratory
in the Development of Joint Laboratory Services." Thesis for the Diploma in Hospital
Administration, University of Toronto.

Fuller, Colleen. 1998. *Caring for Profit: How Corporations Are Taking Over Canada's
Health Care System.* Vancouver: New Star Books.

_____. 1999. "Partnering for Profit, Undermining Medicare: A Comprehensive
Investigation of MDS Inc." British Columbia: Hospital Employees Union.

Gamble, Brenda. 2002. "The Commercialization of Hospital-Based Medical Laboratory
Services: A Comparative Case Study in Ontario Documenting and Analyzing the
Implication for Patients, Providers and the Health Care System." Master of Science
thesis, Graduate Department of the Institute of Medical Sciences, University of
Toronto.

Gibbs, Lennox, and Esam El-Makkawy. 2009. "CML Healthcare Income Fund: U.S.
Imaging Volumes Resilient — Q2/09 Review." Equity Research from Newcrest, a
Division of TD Securities Inc., Toronto, August 12.

Globe and Mail. 1977a. "ABKO Lab Gave Dr. Tse Kickbacks: Court Told." February 2.

_____. 1977b. "Small Towns Will be Hurt by Lab Law, OMA Says." May 11.

_____. 1977c. "Ziemba Jailed for Refusing to Name Sources in ABKO Lab Fraud Case."
June 24.

Gold, G., P.J. Plant, and H.I. MacKillop. 1979. "Review of the Salient Features of the
Ontario Laboratory Industry and Policy Options." Ministry of Health internal document, July 20. Archives of Ontario, RG 10-39, Box 3, B167577.

Goozner, Merrill. 2004. *The $800 Million Dollar Pill: The Truth Behind the Cost of New
Drugs.* Berkley: University of California Press.

Gould, Paul. 1997. "Integrated Delivery Systems: OAML Perspective on Funding." CEO
of the OAML, speech to the CLMA Trillium Chapter, April 16.

Greenwood, John. 1999. "Interest in Med-Chem Simmers as Deadline Looms." *Financial
Post* March 10.

GSA Consulting Group Inc. 1993. "The Establishment of a Centralized Database and
Electronic Communication Links for Laboratory Data." Laboratory Services Review,
Ontario Ministry of Health.

Hadler, Nortin. 2004. *The Last Well Person: How to Stay Well Despite the Health-Care*

System. Montreal: McGill-Queen's University Press.

Hamilton Spectator. 2002. "Healthy Takeover Deal for GDML." May 10.

Harding, Katherine. 2002. "Toronto's Dynacare to Be Taken Over by Labcorp of America in $1B Deal." *Canadian Press* May 9.

HICL. 1981. "Supplement #2: Report of the Chairman of the Board and President to the Annual General Meeting, June 3, 1981: Historical Account." Don Mills: Hospitals In-Common Laboratory Inc.

Information and Privacy Commissioner. 1994. "Order PO-665, Appeal P-9300610." April 15. <ipc.on.ca/scripts/index_.asp?action=31&P_ID=4935&N_ID1&PT_ID=2233>.

_____. 2003. "Order PO-2145, Appeal PA-020292-1." May 20. <accessandprivacy.gov.on.ca/english/order/prov/PO-2145.htm>.

IPSOS Canada. 2006. "Canadians on Healthcare." Media release, January 18.

Jentz, L.A. 1968. "Some Aspects of Laboratory Centralization." A paper presented to the OMA section on Clinical Pathology, May 10. Archives of Ontario, RG 10-247, container 1, B134859.

Kilshaw, Miles, et al. 1992. "Review of Diagnostic Laboratory Services: A Report to the Minister of Health Province of Saskatchewan."

Korstrom Glen. 2010. "Goodreau Finds Life After LifeLabs: Multiple CEO Roles and Board Posts Mean Her Options for the Future Are Wide Open." *Business in Vancouver* March 23–29. <biv.com/iwib/2010/i-ida.asp>.

LabCorp. 2009. *LabCorp, Laboratory Corporation of America: 2009 Annual Report.*

Lang, Michelle. 2009. "Critics Raise Lab Contract Concern: Health Board Executive Is Former Worker of Winning Firm." *Calgary Herald* Jun 19.

Leys, Colin. 2001. *Market-Driven Politics: Neo-liberal Democracy and the Public Interest.* London: Verso.

_____. 2009. "Health, Heath Care and Capitalism." In Leo Panitch and Colin Leys (eds.), *Morbid Symptoms: Health Under Capitalism.* London: Merlin Press.

Marriot, John. 1993. "Review of Laboratory Services Funding: Background/Discussion Paper." Laboratory Services Review, Ontario Ministry of Health.

McIntosh, Tom, and Michael Ducie. 2009. "Private Health Facilities in Saskatchewan: Marginalization Through Legalization." *Canadian Political Science Review* 3,4 (December).

McQueen, M.J., and A.J. Bailey. 1993a. "A Cost Accounting Prototype in the Clinical Laboratory: The Hamilton Health Sciences Laboratory Program." *Clinical Diagnostics Today* March.

_____. 1993b. "Hamilton Health Sciences Laboratory Program: A Provider Developed Model for Hospital, University and Community Services." *Healthcare Management Forum* 6, 3 (Fall/Autumn).

MDS. 2005. *Focused on High Growth Life Science Markets: MDS 2005 Annual Report.*

Ministère de la Santé et des Services Sociaux. 2008. "Tableaux de Bord de Gestion des Laboratoires de Biologie Médicale Année Financière 2006–2007." Gouvernement du Québec. ISBN: 978-2-550-53629-1 (version PDF)

Mittelstaedt, Martin. 2010. "Some Provinces Getting a Bad Deal on Vitamin D Tests." *Globe and Mail* January 20.

More, David. 1994. "Bang for the Buck: Alternatives for Funding Ontario in Funding Medical Laboratory Services." Project for Master of Public Administration, Queen's University.

_____. 2006/2007. "Testing for Profit: Lab Work by Private Corporation Hides Behind Not-for-Profit Clinic." *Independent Voice* December/January.

More, David, Sandip Sengupta, and Paul Manley. 2000. "Promoting, Building and Sustaining a Regional Laboratory Network in a Changing Environment." *Clinical Leadership & Management Review* 14,5 (September/October).

Nicol, John, and Stephanie Nolen. 1998. "Canada: The Battle for Medicare Cash: Health-Care Firms Seek to Protect their Market Share as Governments Cut Back." *Maclean's* January 6.

Office of the Auditor General of Ontario. 2005. *2005 Annual Report.* Toronto: Queen's Printer.

Ontario Association of Medical Laboratories. 2003. "The SARS Outbreak in Ontario, 2003: The Community Laboratory Perspective." Toronto: OAML.

Ontario Council of Health. 1982. *Report of the Task Force on Laboratory Services.* Ontario Ministry of Health.

Ontario Health Coalition. 2010. "Toward Access and Quality: Realigning Ontario's Approach to Small and Rural Hospitals to Serve Public Values, Results of the Ontario Health Coalition Hearings on Small and Rural Hospitals held in 12 Communities Across Ontario." May 17. Toronto.

Ontario Hospital Association. 1994. "Response to Laboratory Services Review External Advisory Sub-Committee Social Contract Study Summary Report." Toronto.

_____. 2000. "Laboratory Service System Issues for Ontario: An Ontario Hospital Association Discussion Paper on Laboratory Services in Ontario." Toronto.

Ontario Hospital e-Health Council: Hospital Laboratory Information Systems Advisory Group. 2006. "Laboratory Information System Integration: A Survey of Current and Proposed Local or Region Models of Connectivity." Toronto: Ontario Hospital Association.

Ontario Medical Review. 1964. "Report of Committee on Tariff." 31.

_____. 1965. "Report of Committee on Tariff." 32.

_____. 1969. "PSI: Abuse of Labs Being Studied." June.

Ontario Ministry of Health. 1974. "Minister Announces New Laboratory Proficiency Testing Program." News release. October 2.

_____. 1976. "Report of the Laboratory Study Committee." September 15. Archives of Ontario, RG 10-39.

_____. 1978. "Minster Announces Control for Medically Unnecessary Laboratory Tests." News release. January 30.

_____. 1979. "Laboratory Program Announced for Kenora and Rainy River Districts." News release. October 10.

_____. 1993a. "Laboratory Services Review Discussion Paper #2: System."

_____. 1993b. "Laboratory Services Review Discussion Paper #3, Human Resources."

_____. 1993c. "Health Service Companies Get Competitive Edge in International Marketplace." News release. November 16.

_____. 1993d. "Ontario Association of Medical Laboratories/Ministry of Health: Memorandum of Understanding." Signed December 17.

_____. 1993e. "Laboratory Services Discussion Paper #1: Utilization."

_____. 1994a. *Laboratory Services Review.*

_____. 1994b. "Study on Costs and Implications of Transferring Laboratory Workload." Laboratory Services Review.

_____. 1996. "Planning Objectives: Laboratory Service Restructuring." June.

_____. n.d. "Laboratory Out-Patient Pilot Project: Evaluation Committee Report." Personal communication. This report is undated and the version I have is a copy of one released after a FOI request. It contains blacked-out sections.

Page, John S., and Barbara Kornovski. 2000. "Provincial Group on Laboratory Reform." Ontario Ministry of Health, June 29.

Parker, James. 1996. "Fewer Medical Lab Workers to Lose Jobs Than First Thought." *Saskatoon Star Phoenix* May 11.

Perry, Tony. 1996. Lab to Pay $182 Million in Fraud Case: Court: Settlement Resolves Charges that LabCorp Billed Medicare, Medicaid and Insurance Programs for Unneeded Tests. A Subsidiary Agrees to a $5-million Criminal Fine." *Los Angeles Times* November 22.

Plain, Richard. 2000. "The Commercialization and Privatization of Hospital Based Medical Services Within the Province of Alberta: A Public Interest Perspective." Medicare Economics Group, Department of Economics, University of Alberta. March.

Plant, Paul. 1977a. "Briefing Material for Minister's Meeting with Ontario Association of Medical Laboratories." September 19. Archives of Ontario, RG 10-39, file: Administration — Ministerial Speeches and Tours, 1977, 52.03.01.

_____. 1977b. "Monopoly Potential in Private Laboratories in Ontario." Ontario Ministry of Health, September 28. Archives of Ontario, RG 10-39, file: Legislation. Monopoly Studies.

Plebani, Mario. 1999. "The Clinical Importance of Laboratory Reasoning." *Clinica Chimica Acta* 280.

Pollard, Alan. 1975. "The In-Common Laboratory, Toronto." *Clinical Biochemistry* 8.

Prashad, Sharda. 2005. "MDS Inc. to Cut Half of Business Units, Slash 550 Jobs." *Globe and Mail* September 2.

Priest, Lisa. 1996. "MDS Cited for Fraud: Some 100 Probed over Kickbacks and Referral Fees." *Toronto Star* February 27.

Pritzker, H.G. 1957. "Provision and Payment of Diagnostic Services: A Symposium: A Pathologists Viewpoint." *Canadian Journal of Public Health* 48 (October).

QMP-LS. 2008. "Ontario Medical Association, Quality Management Program — Laboratory Services, 2008 Annual Review." Toronto.

QSE Consulting. 2006. "Third Party Review of the Eastern Ontario Regional Laboratory Association's Business Case: Final Report." Toronto: Queens Printer for Ontario.

Rempel, Shauna. 2004. "Health Region Contract Irks Union: New Service Provider Not Unionized." *Saskatoon Star Phoenix* January 21.

RPO Management Consultants. 2008. "Laboratory Pilot Projects Review: Final Report." Ontario Ministry of Health, March 31.

Sack Goldblatt Mitchell LLP, Lawyers. 2008. "Re: Eastern Ontario Laboratory Association and Gamma-Dynacare Medical Laboratories." A legal opinion written for the Ontario Council of Hospital Unions, Toronto. October 31.

Saskatchewan Health. 1991. "Comparative Costs of Laboratory Services." February 20. Report attached to a letter from Glenda Yeats, Associate Deputy Minister, Saskatchewan Health to the Saskatchewan Medical Association, February 21, 1991.

_____. 2009. "Medical Services Branch: Annual Statistical Report 08–09."

Simpson, Jim. 1999. "Ontario Courts Dismiss Further Challenges to Gov't Management of the Health Care System." *Ontario Medical Review* November 1.

Sinnema, Jodie. 2010. "Centralized Lab Test Bad Idea: Pathologists." *Edmonton Journal* February 19.

Skerritt, Jen. 2009. "Overwork in DSM Labs Leads to Concerns About Quality, Diagnostic Flaws a Danger: MD." *Winnipeg Free Press* December 11.

St. Pierre, Denis. 1996. "Officials Deny Conflict in MDs Proposal." *Sudbury Star* March 4.

Sutherland, Jim. 2004. "Unbeatable: Even After Cuts in Funding, BC Biomedical Is Our No. 1 Employer for the Third Year in a Row. Here's How They Do It." *Globe and Mail* December 24.

Sutherland, Ross. 2007. "Biting the Hand That Feeds You: The Political Economy of Ontario's Community Laboratory Services." Master of Arts thesis, Institute of Political Economy, Carleton University, Ottawa, Ontario.

Swartz, Donald. 1977. "The Politics of Reform: Conflict and Accommodation in Canadian Health Policy." In Leo Panitch (ed.), *The Canadian State: Political Economy and Political Power.* Toronto: University of Toronto Press.

Taylor, Malcolm. 1978. *Health Insurance and Canadian Public Policy: The Seven Decisions that Created the Canadian Health Insurance System.* Montreal: McGill-Queen's University Press.

Thorburn, Michael. 1999. "Ontario Laboratory Industry in Transition Prompts Physician Concern: Access to Patient Services, Revised Practice Arrangements among Issues Cited." *Ontario Medical Review* 60, 5 (May).

Times-Colonist. 2009. "Lab Errors Show Lack of Oversight." Victoria, June 7.

Toronto Star. 1999. "GDML Medical Laboratories." April 7.

Twohig, Peter L. 2005. *Labour in the Laboratory: Medical Laboratory Workers in the Maritimes, 1900–1950.* Montreal: McGill-Queen's University Press.

Valorzi, John. 2007. "MDS Share Buyback Wins Board Approval." *Globe and Mail* February 27.

Van Walraven, Carl, Goel Vivek and Ben Chan. 1998. "Effect of Population-based Interventions on Laboratory Utilization: A Time-Series Analysis." *JAMA* 280, 230 (December 16).

Verbugge, R. 1972. "An Explanatory Memorandum on the Federal Cost Sharing Formula." Internal Ministry of Health document. Archives of Ontario, RG 10-221-2, box 40, B394786, file: 497.

Waldie, Paul. 1996. "MDS Predicts Profit Rise: Firm Has Broadened Range of Services." *Globe and Mail* March 20.

Walkom, Thomas. 1994. "Kickbacks to Doctors Would be Headache for NDP." *Toronto Star* July 28.

Watts, Michael. 1997. "Laboratory Restructuring in Ontario." *Hospital News* February.

Yalnizyan, Armine. 2004. "Can We Afford to Sustain Medicare? A Strong Role for Federal Government." Ottawa: Canadian Federation of Nurses Unions.

Zehr, Leonard. 2005. "New Leader, New Life for Tired MDS." *Globe and Mail* August 20.
_____. 2006. "MDS Reaps Windfall with $1.3-Billion Sale of Lab Unit. "*Globe and Mail* October 6.

Acknowledgements

The research for this study would not have been possible without public funding from the Graduate Student Scholarship and Carleton University, which allowed me to take time off work to do the initial research that laid the groundwork for this book. My employer, Street Health, gave me time off to do further research and write the book.

The information gathered depended upon the generous input of dozens of individuals, many of whom do not wish to be named. The heated politics of laboratory delivery make disclosure uncomfortable for some, so to all of you, thank you for helping out.

I would specifically like to thank Andy Summers, Dave More, Frank Nasca, Pete Hudson, Kathleen Connors, Marie Claude Premont, Elisabeth Ballerman, Celine Castonguay, Colleen Fuller, Guillaume Hebert and Wendy Armstrong for assistance with research and comments on early drafts.

Special thanks goes to my father, Dr. Ralph Sutherland, who provided invaluable text suggestions, and my mother, Dr. Eleanor Sutherland, who, still practising medicine at eighty-two, fed me wonderful leads on the impact of for-profit laboratories on her daily work. Hugh Armstrong, my thesis advisor, told me to concentrate on the story and provided many comments on drafts. Candida Hadley at Fernwood Press reinforced this message and provided great guidance. Pamela Martin was invaluable with timely editing help.

Finally, I would like to thank Nancy Bayly, the love of my life, who tolerated endless disruptions to our life, and my granddaughter Brianna, who did not understand why I wanted to write about medical laboratories but encouraged me by being thrilled that I was writing a book.

As valuable as all this help was I take full responsibility for the final synthesis, and any errors in the text are my own.

NEW in the Basic Series
from Fernwood Publishing

Sex and the Supreme Court
Obscenity and Indecency Law in Canada

Richard Jochelson & Kirsten Kramar

9781552664155 $17.95 112pp Rights: World May 2011

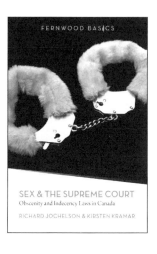

Canadian laws pertaining to pornography and bawdy houses
were first developed during the Victorian era, when "non-
normative" sexualities were understood as a corruption
of conservative morals and harmful to society as a whole.
Tracing the socio-legal history of contemporary obscenity and
indecency laws, Kramar and Jochelson contend that the law
continues to function to protect society from harm. Today, rather
than seeing harm to conservative values, the court sees harm to
liberal political values. While reforms have been made, especially
in light of feminist and queer challenges, Kramar and Jochelson
use Foucault's governmentality framework to show that the
liberal harm strategy for governing obscenity and indecency continues to disguise power.

RICHARD JOCHELSON is a professor of criminal justice at the University of Winnipeg. KIRSTEN
KRAMAR is a professor of sociology at the University of Winnipeg.

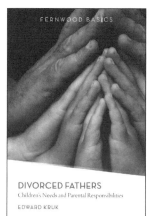

Divorced Fathers
Children's Needs and Parental Responsibilities

Edward Kruk

9781552664087 $17.95 128pp Rights: World May 2011

Once mainly breadwinners and disciplinarians, fathers are
becoming increasingly involved and invested in their children's
lives. Edward Kruk examines how this changing role has affected
fathers' experiences of divorce and the loss of children that too
often follows. This book offers a glimpse into the emotional
loss that fathers suffer and their perspectives on what is best
for their children in the divorce transition. Ultimately, Kruk
argues, children benefit most from the love and support of both
parents, and we need to ensure that fathers continue to play a
meaningful parenting role after divorce.

EDWARD KRUK is an associate professor of social work at
University of British Columbia. He is the author of *Mediation and Conflict Resolution in Social Work
and Human Services* (1997) and *Divorce and Disengagement: Patterns of Fatherhood Within and
Beyond Marriage* (1993).

visit www.fernwoodpublishing.ca for the complete list of the Basics Series